:😊: —A true em_____cy, _ outlined above. Memorizing these conditions may help, rather than referring to this book when the patient is in the department! Call for immediate senior help. Try to remain calm and quickly assess the ABCs. Once the problem has been dealt with, remember to re-assess— other problems may have been forgotten or missed in the heat of the moment.

:😐: —These patients still need to be assessed very quickly, but you do not need to drop everything and run (so long as their ABCs have been managed). These patients can quickly shift into the emergency category if not sorted soon. Consider senior help/advise.

① The majority of patients will fall into this and the last category. Although they do not need to be seen straight away, make sure you assess ___ thoroughly—some conditions can deteriorate if not treated properly. Think carefully of potential complications that may develop, such as ___ ventricular block with inferior MIs or tamponade with pericardial ___ns. Liaise with specialist help, if necessary.

⑦ – ___ are non urgent conditions and general points of interest. ___y o: patients, strictly speaking, should not come to casualty in ___irst

OXFORD MEDICAL PUBLICATIONS

Emergencies in Cardiology

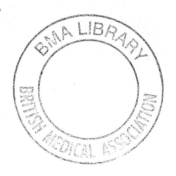

Emergencies in Cardiology

Edited by

Saul G. Myerson

Clinical Lecturer in Cardiovascular Medicine,
University of Oxford, Oxford, UK

Robin P. Choudhury

Clinical Lecturer in Cardiovascular Medicine,
University of Oxford, Oxford, UK

Andrew R. J. Mitchell

Specialist Registrar in Cardiology,
John Radcliffe Hospital, Oxford, UK

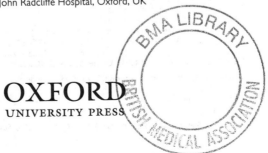

OXFORD
UNIVERSITY PRESS

OXFORD
UNIVERSITY PRESS

Great Clarendon Street, Oxford OX2 6DP

Oxford University Press is a department of the University of Oxford.
It furthers the University's objective of excellence in research, scholarship,
and education by publishing worldwide in

Oxford New York

Auckland Cape Town Dar es Salaam Hong Kong Karachi
Kuala Lumpur Madrid Melbourne Mexico City Nairobi
New Delhi Shanghai Taipei Toronto

With offices in

Argentina Austria Brazil Chile Czech Republic France Greece
Guatemala Hungary Italy Japan Poland Portugal Singapore
South Korea Switzerland Thailand Turkey Ukraine Vietnam

Oxford is a registered trade mark of Oxford University Press
in the UK and in certain other countries

Published in the United States
by Oxford University Press Inc., New York

© Oxford University Press 2006

A catalogue record for this title is available from the British Library

Library of Congress Cataloging in Publication Data
Oxford handbook of emergencies in cardiology/edited by Saul G. Myerson, Robin P.
Choudhury, Andrew Mitchell.— 1ˢᵗ ed.
Includes bibliographical references and index.
1. Cardiovascular emergencies–Handbooks, manuals, etc. [DNLM: 1. Cardiovascular
Diseases–Handbooks.   2. Emergencies–Handbooks. WG 39 O98 2006] I. Title: Handbook
of emergencies in cardiology.   II. Myerson, Saul G.   III. Choudhury, Robin P.   IV.
Mitchell, Andrew, 1968-RC675.O94 2006 616.1'025–dc22 2005022018

Typeset by Newgen Imaging Systems (P) Ltd., Chennai, India
Printed in Italy
on acid-free paper by
LegoPrint S.p.A

ISBN 0–19–856959–9 (flexicover: alk. paper)   978–0–19–856959–6 (flexicover: alk. paper)

10 9 8 7 6 5 4 3 2 1

Foreword

This pocket-sized book (for a largeish pocket) is aimed at physicians in training as a *vade mecum* to help them make a sensible assessment of patients presenting with symptoms of the common cardiac emergencies—chest pain, breathlessness, syncope, palpitations etc.

The authors succeed brilliantly in their task. The style is terse, authoritative and didactic, but web links are given for further information. The text throughout uses familiar abbreviations—CXR, STEMI, ICD, SK etc. (but provides an explanatory list of all abbreviations).

Each chapter conforms to a standard format and avoids the problems and variable quality which is often found in a multi-author text. Unlike standard textbooks of cardiology (usually written by senior figures), this book is clearly written by (and for) those who meet these conditions early in their evolution. The book is a distillation of up-to-date first-hand experience, full of wisdom and tempered by very practical advice on how to avoid the complications of too aggressive treatment.

The initial 5 chapters are concerned with the rapid evaluation and differential diagnosis of cardiovascular collapse (arrest/shock), chest pain, shortness of breath, syncope, and palpitation; these take the form of lists of specific things to elucidate from the history and examination. The immediate actions and emergency investigations are then listed, followed by recommendations for emergency treatment. The lists are concise, with (on each line) very useful and clear cross-referencing to the pages in the book where the reader can find the likely differential diagnosis or details of procedures or treatment, such as CPAP, echocardiography. Then follow chapters on specific emergency conditions such as acute coronary syndromes, acute heart failure, cardiogenic shock, and all the gamut of acute cardiology.

The book ends with excellent chapters on practical procedures—cardiotoxic drugs, overdose of cardiovascular drugs. Finally a chapter on ECGs illustrates both common and uncommon (Brugada) tracings relevant to emergency cardiology.

This book fills a much needed niche. It will be of great benefit to busy and worried house staff and registrars—in both cardiology and internal medicine. It will also be helpful in general practice, as it is both concise and very user-friendly.

Professor Peter Sleight
Hon Consultant Cardiologist
Professor Emeritus of Cardiovascular Medicine
John Radcliffe Hospital
University of Oxford

Preface

Cardiac emergencies are some of the most alarming and exciting medical conditions facing both the experienced front-line emergency room physician and the most junior ward doctor. They are an extremely common cause of hospital admission and also frequently occur in medical and surgical in-patients. A diagnosis and management plan must be made quickly, guided by knowledge and experience. The principal aim of this book is to aid this with expert advice in a clear, concise format using the familiar Oxford Handbook style.

The first section of the book is symptom based and entitled 'Presentation – making the diagnosis'. This section is designed to help clinch the diagnosis with suggestions of the key points in the history, physical findings, and investigations. There is extensive cross-referencing to specific cardiac conditions later in the book.

The second section 'Specific conditions' describes the presentation, investigation, and management of all the common (and some uncommon) acute cardiac problems. The chapter authors have used their specialist knowledge to present the relevant vital diagnostic steps and early management plans. This section also includes chapters on important cardiology problems in which specialist advice is vital but often not immediately available. This includes sections on the management of potentially challenging problems such as arrhythmias (and implantable defibrillators), cardiac issues in pregnancy, management of cardiac problems around the time of surgery, emergencies in adults with congenital heart disease, and the management of cardiac trauma.

The final section deals with 'practical issues', with clear descriptions of how to perform common practical cardiac procedures. It also includes a chapter on the art of ECG recognition with a library of example ECGs to help pattern recognition.

We hope that you enjoy the book and use it to enhance the care of your patients. We welcome suggestions for alterations and inclusions in future editions. A 'comments card' is provided for this purpose or you can contact us via the OUP website: http://www.oup.co.uk

The Editors
2005

Contents

Contributors *xi*

Symbols and abbreviations *xiii*

Presentation—making the diagnosis

1	Cardiovascular collapse	**3**
2	Chest pain	**15**
3	Shortness of breath	**21**
4	Syncope	**27**
5	Palpitation	**37**

Specific conditions

6	Acute coronary syndromes	**45**
7	Acute heart failure	**67**
8	Valve disease	**87**
9	Arrhythmias	**125**
10	Aortic dissection	**169**
11	Pericardial disease	**181**
12	Pulmonary vascular disease	**189**
13	Systemic emboli	**201**
14	Cardiac issues in pregnancy	**207**
15	Adult congenital heart disease	**217**
16	Peri-operative care	**247**
17	Cardiotoxic drug overdose	**261**
18	Miscellaneous conditions	**277**

Practical issues

19	Practical procedures	**287**
20	ECG recognition	**305**

Index *343*

Contents

Contributors

Adrian Banning
Consultant Cardiologist
John Radcliffe Hospital, Oxford
Aortic dissection

Harald Becher
Consultant Cardiologist
John Radcliffe Hospital, Oxford
Pericardial disease

Tim Betts
Consultant Cardiologist
John Radcliffe Hospital, Oxford
Arrhythmias
Acute coronary syndromes

Keith Channon
Professor of Cardiovascular Medicine
Oxford University, Oxford
Acute coronary syndromes

Robin Choudhury
Clinical Lecturer in Cardiovascular
  Medicine
Oxford University, Oxford
Chest pain
Acute coronary syndromes

Jeremy Dwight
Consultant Cardiologist
John Radcliffe Hospital, Oxford
Heart failure

Pierre Foex
Professor of Anaesthetics
Oxford University, Oxford
Peri-operative issues

Andrew Mitchell
Specialist Registrar in Cardiology
John Radcliffe Hospital, Oxford
Shortness of breath
Syncope
Aortic dissection
Pulmonary vascular disease
Miscellaneous conditions

Steve Murray
Consultant Cardiologist
Middlesborough General Hospital
ECG recognition

Saul Myerson
Clinical Lecturer in Cardiovascular
  Medicine
Oxford University, Oxford
Palpitation
Valve disease

Mark Petersen
Consultant Cardiologist
Gloucester Royal Hospital
Syncope

Jonathan Salmon
Consultant in Intensive Care
  Medicine
John Radcliffe Hospital, Oxford
Cardiovascular collapse

Cheerag Shirodaria
Specialist Registrar in Cardiology
John Radcliffe Hospital, Oxford
Cardiotoxic drug overdose

Rod Stables
Consultant Cardiologist
The Cardiothoracic Centre,
Liverpool
Practical procedures

Sara Thorne
Consultant Cardiologist
University Hospital,
   Birmingham
Cardiac issues in pregnancy

Jonathan Timperley
Specialist Registrar in Cardiology
John Radcliffe Hospital, Oxford
Emboli

Anselm Uebing
Anna John
Michael Gatzoulis
Adult Congenital Heart Disease Unit
Royal Brompton Hospital, London
Adult congenital heart disease

Symbols and abbreviations

❶	Warning
⚠	Warning
📖	Cross-reference
►	Important
►►	Don't dawdle
△△	Differential diagnosis
↓	Decreased
↑	Increased
↔	Normal
1°	Primary
2°	Secondary
ACC	American College of Cardiologists
ACE	Angiotensin converting enzyme
ACS	Acute coronary syndrome
AHA	American Heart Association
AF	Atrial fibrillation
ANA	Anti-nuclear antibodies
Apo	Apolipoprotein
AR	Aortic regurgitation
ARDS	Adult respiratory distress syndrome
AS	Aortic stenosis
ASD	Atrial septal defect
AV	Atrioventricular
AVR	Aortic valve replacement
AVNRT	Atrioventricular nodal re-entrant tachycardia
AVRT	Atrioventricular re-entrant tachycardia
BBB	Bundle branch block
BiPAP	Bilevel positive pressure support
BNP	Brain natriuretic peptide
BP	Blood pressure
CCU	Coronary care unit
CHB	Complete (3rd degree) heart block
CK	Creatine kinase
CT	Computerised tomography
COPD	Chronic obstructive pulmonary disease
CPAP	Continuous positive airways pressure
CPR	Cardiopulmonary resuscitation

CRP	C reactive protein
CT	Computed tomography
CXR	Chest X-ray
DIC	Disseminated intravascular coagulation
dsDNA	Double stranded DNA
DVT	Deep vein thrombosis
ECG	Electrocardiogram
FBC	Full blood count
GpIIbIIIa	Glycoprotein IIb IIIa
GTN	Glyceryl tri-nitrate
GUSTO	Global Utilization of Streptokinase and t-PA for Occluded Coronary Arteries
HCM	Hypertrophic cardiomyopathy
HDL	High density lipoproteins
HbO2	Oxygenated haemoglobin
ICD	Implantable cardioverter defibrillator
ITU	Intensive therapy unit
IVC	Inferior vena cava
JVP	Jugular venous pressure
LAD	Left anterior descending coronary artery
LBBB	Left bundle branch block
LCX	Circumflex coronary artery
LDH	Lactate dehydrogenase
LDL	Low density lipoproteins
LV	Left ventricle
LVH	Left ventricular hypertrophy
MI	Myocardial infarction
MR	Mitral regurgitation
MRI	Magnetic resonance imaging
NSAID	Non-steroidal anti-inflammatory drug
NSTEMI	Non-ST-segment elevation MI
PCI	Percutaneous coronary intervention
PDA	Patent ductus arteriosus
PE	Pulmonary embolism
PFO	Patent foramen ovale
RBBB	Right bundle branch block
RCA	Right coronary artery
rt-PA	Recombinant tissue plasminogen activator
RV	Right ventricle
SK	Streptokinase
STEMI	ST elevation myocardial infarction
SVT	Supraventricular tachycardia
TIMI	Thrombolysis in myocardial infarction (clinical trial)

TNK	Tenecteplase
TOE	Transoesophageal echocardiography
TTE	Transthoracic echocardiography
UA	Unstable angina
U&E	Urea and electrolytes
VT	Ventricular tachycardia
VF	Ventricular fibrillation
VQ	Ventilation perfusion
VSD	Ventricular septal defect
VTE	Venous thromboembolism

Presentation—making the diagnosis

Cardiovascular collapse

Cardiovascular collapse 4
Cardiac arrest 4
Shock 4
Initial assessment 6
Approaching a differential in shock 6
Causes of shock 7
Immediate actions 8
Continuing investigation and treatment 10

Cardiovascular collapse

Cardiovascular collapse is the rapid or sudden development of circulatory failure. This forms part of a spectrum which encompasses:
- Cardiac arrest
- Shock—overt and compensated.

☠ Cardiac arrest

Treat immediately according to current guidelines (see opposite).

✚ Shock

Systolic BP <90 mmHg with features of reduced organ perfusion.

In shock, cardiac output may be high (e.g. sepsis) or low (e.g. cardiogenic shock). The common factor is failure of tissue oxygen delivery and/or tissue oxygen utilisation. The clinical presentation depends upon the severity and speed of onset of the cause and the physiologic reserve of the host. Determining the cause may be difficult and the diagnosis may only be apparent following, or during, resuscitation. Pathologies frequently co-exist, particularly in the elderly (e.g. cardiac failure complicating sepsis).

▶ Assessment and treatment should proceed in parallel.

The immediate priorities are to maintain:
- A safe airway and oxygenation
- Sufficient circulation to perfuse the heart and brain.

When these have been achieved, there is time to refine the diagnosis and indulge in special investigations and specific treatment while continuing to resuscitate the circulation.

This may involve a trade-off between giving fluids and vasoactive drugs to improve the peripheral circulation at the expense of increasing myocardial work. However, it is critical: failure to restore adequate tissue perfusion vastly increases mortality and makes all your hard work meaningless.

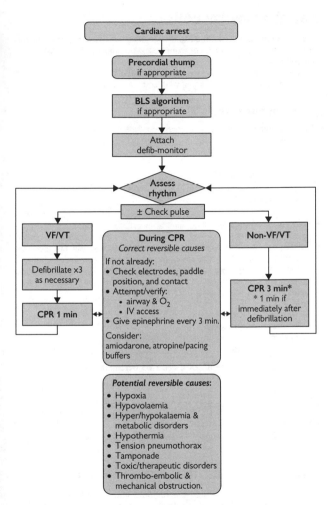

The Advanced Life Support universal algorithm for the management of cardiac arrest in adults.

Initial assessment

This should be rapid. You need to decide whether the patient can survive more detailed assessment or whether you must start resuscitating immediately.

▶ If the patient can speak, take a brief, focused history. If not, assess the patient whilst questioning nursing staff, ambulance personnel or relatives.

Check immediately

- Airway competence
- Breathing
- Circulation—pulse: rate and character.

Specifically examine

- Peripheral perfusion, including capillary refill
- Blood pressure
- JVP
- Is there a sternotomy scar?
- Check the trachea
- Percuss the upper chest and listen to air entry to exclude pneumothorax and for crackles of pulmonary oedema
- Listen to the heart. Are there any (possibly new) murmurs?
- Quickly feel the abdomen for distension, pulsatile masses etc.
- Assess conscious level using the AVPU score:
  - A = awake
  - V = responds to voice only
  - P = responds to pain
  - U= unresponsive
- Check capillary blood sugar.

Obtain (or nominate a colleague to obtain)

- 12-lead ECG
- Chest X-ray
- Arterial blood gas analysis
- Urgent biochemistry (U&E, Ca^{2+}, Mg^{2+}, troponin, glucose, CK, amylase)
- FBC, clotting studies, group and save
- If sepsis seems likely, check CRP and send blood cultures.

Approaching a differential in shock

At the end of this you should have sufficient information to make a preliminary diagnosis and assign the patient to one of three main categories:
- Intrinsic cardiogenic
- Extrinsic 'cardiogenic'
- Non-cardiogenic.

See box opposite for causes.

Causes of shock

Intrinsic cardiogenic
- Acute myocardial failure
- Acute myocardial ischaemia
- Acute valvular lesion
- Cardio-depressant drugs
- Arrhythmia.

Extrinsic 'cardiogenic'
- Pulmonary embolus
- Pericardial tamponade
- Tension pneumothorax.

Non-cardiogenic
- Sepsis
- Anaphylaxis
- Hypovolaemia
- Vasoactive drug toxicity (drug-induced hypotension).

Immediate actions

▶ Reassess Airway, Breathing, Circulation frequently.

▶ ☼ Treat cardiac arrest according to protocol.

Initial targets
- Mean arterial blood pressure >60 mmHg (systolic >90 mmHg)
- PaO_2 >8 kPa.

Respiratory management
- ☼ Place Guedel airway if patient unconscious to maintain airway
- High-flow O_2 via reservoir bag or assist ventilation with bag and mask
- ☼ For tension pneumothorax perform immediate needle thoracostomy followed by formal chest drainage
- If the patient is conscious, hypoxic and has pulmonary oedema or respiratory distress, face-mask continuous airways pressure (CPAP 📖 p.10) may be a valuable precursor or alternative to intubation.

When to call the anaesthetist
- Airway compromised
- Severe respiratory failure:
  - Respiratory rate >30 or <10
  - PaO_2 <10 on high-flow oxygen
  - ↑$PaCO_2$
- Patient comatose (AVPU = P or U)
- Cardioversion likely to be required
- Do not attempt intubation without good IV access and resuscitation drugs, unless patient is already in cardiac arrest.

Circulatory management
- Establish good peripheral IV access
- If significant bradycardia, give atropine 0.5–1 mg IV and consider external pacing if inadequate response (📖 p.296)
- If the patient is not in intrinsic cardiogenic shock and is without evidence of intravascular volume overload or pulmonary oedema, give rapid IV fluid challenge (100–200 mL colloid or 250–500 mL Hartmann's/0.9% saline). If beneficial, repeat
- If blood pressure remains low (<70 mmHg systolic) despite adequate filling and treatment of immediately reversible causes, obtain central venous access and start inotropes (see box opposite)
- If there are delays in obtaining central venous access or in setting up an infusion of inotropes, consider small boluses of epinephrine (0.25–0.5 mL 1:10,000 from a Minijet®) peripherally. Remember, circulation time will be long: there may be no response for 60 seconds (it will feel longer).

General management
- If glucose low, give 50 mL, 50% dextrose immediately
- If pupils are constricted and patient is unresponsive, give naloxone 200–400 mcg IV stat. If improvement, repeat.

Table of inotropes

	Formulation	Dose range	Initial dose (70 kg man)
VASODILATORS			
GTN			
Initial treatment of angina or acute LVF	Bolus (sublingual spray)	500 mcg	2–4 puffs
Continued treatment of angina or LVF	Infusion 1 mg/mL	50 mg in 50 mL 0.9% saline	0.5–20 mg/h	2–5 mL/h
INODILATORS			
Dobutamine	Infusion 5 mg/mL	250 mg in 50 mL 0.9% saline	1.25–10 mcg/kg/min	1.6–4 mL/h (approx 2–5 mcg/kg/min)
INOCONSTRICTORS			
Epinephrine			
In extremis	Bolus (minijet)	1 mg in 10 mL	p.r.n.	0.5 mL bolus
Increase BP and cardiac output	Infusion	4 mg in 50 mL 0.9% saline	Up to 50 mL/h (titrate to effect)	2–5 mL/h
Dopamine As epinephrine	Infusion	200 mg in 50 mL 0.9% saline	1–10 mcg/kg/min	2–5 mL/h (approx 2–5 mcg/kg/min)
Ephedrine As epinephrine Slower onset (2–10 min) and longer lasting	Bolus 3 mg/mL	Dilute 30 mg (1 mL) to 10 mL with 0.9% saline		1 mL of dilute solution
VASOCONSTRICTORS			
Norepinephrine 'Pure' vasoconstriction— increase BP, little effect on CO	Infusion	4 mg in 50 mL 0.9% saline	Up to 50 mL/h (titrate to effect)	2–5 mL/h
Metaraminol 'Pure' vasoconstrictor. Slow onset—max effect at 10 mins	Bolus	Dilute 10 mg (1 mL) to 10 mL with 0.9% saline		0.5–5 mL bolus of dilute solution

Infusions should be given centrally. Dopamine and dobutamine can be given peripherally at lower concentrations (dilute in 500 mL, not 50 mL). Caution with extravasation of bolus drugs. An inoconstrictor (epinephrine or dopamine) can be used if norepinephrine is not immediately to hand. Norepinephrine is preferable if the patient is very tachycardic (>120 bpm) or if there is clear evidence of myocardial ischaemia. Ephedrine or metaraminol are reasonable alternatives for peripheral boluses (see table).

Continuing investigation and treatment

If the underlying diagnosis is obvious, you can now initiate definitive treatment. Otherwise, the most useful investigation to perform next is an urgent echocardiogram which will inform on:
- LV dysfunction (MI, myocarditis, cardiomyopathy) 📖 p68
- Wall-motion abnormalities (ischaemia)
- Valvular/structural lesions 📖 p88
- Pericardial disease/tamponade 📖 p184
- Right-sided cardiac dilatation (PE, decompensated pulmonary hypertension) 📖 p.190.

Other investigations might include:
- CT pulmonary angiogram (PE)
- CT thorax/abdomen (aortic/intra-abdominal pathology).

Monitoring and assessment of the circulation

For all conditions, is the circulation adequate?
- Ideally HR 60–100. Higher or lower rates may be acceptable if all other components of the circulation are adequate
- Mean arterial blood pressure (diastolic + pulse pressure/3) should be at least 60 to allow adequate cerebral perfusion. Previously hypertensive patients may require a higher pressure
- Diastolic BP must be sufficient to allow myocardial perfusion (>35–40 mmHg, no ST depression on ECG)
- Urine output >0.5 mL/kg/h
- Capillary refill should be <2 seconds
- Lactate concentration should be <2.0 mmol/L, preferably <1.6. If higher, it should fall in response to resuscitation.

Continuous positive airway pressure (CPAP)

In left ventricular dysfunction, CPAP has pulmonary and cardiac benefits. It increases functional residual capacity, thus increasing the effective alveolar surface area and improving oxygenation and, in most patients, reduces the work of breathing (caution if chest hyper-inflated or restrictive chest-wall disease). Cardiac effects include a reduction in LV preload, improved ejection fraction, and reduction in mitral regurgitation.

Non-invasive ventilation

Non-invasive ventilation is more controversial and should probably not be applied in patients with LV failure. If CPAP is inadequate, it is probably better to intubate the patient and ventilate formally.

Central venous monitoring

Central venous cannulae should be placed by the internal jugular or sub-clavian route into the superior vena cava (not the right atrium) 📖 p.290. This allows monitoring of right-sided filling pressures and the dynamic response to fluid challenges, repeated central venous blood gas estimation (of no value for pO_2 and pCO_2 but useful for tracking changes in pH and [lactate]), and estimation of central venous oxygen saturation ($ScvO_2$).

Central venous pressure

Normal CVP is approximately 4–8 cmH$_2$O and should reflect both right and left ventricular end-diastolic pressures. Changes in circulating vol-ume, venoconstriction or dilatation, and pulmonary vascular disease may all mean that CVP does not reflect left-sided filling pressures.

▶ In all causes of shock, myocardial filling pressures need to increase to maintain stroke volume.

Consequently, static measurement of CVP is of little value and it is better to measure the response to a volume challenge.

Fluid challenge

- The principle is that a fluid challenge will produce an initial rise in CVP but, when the infusion is completed, the fluid will redistribute and the CVP will then fall, particularly in hypovolaemia
- In well-filled patients, there will be a net increase in CVP which will be sustained
- By convention, 200 mL of colloid (500 mL of crystalloid) is given over 10–15 minutes, the CVP is measured before the infusion starts, immediately it is completed and again 10–15 minutes later
- A sustained rise in CVP above baseline of >3 cmH$_2$O indicates the circulation is well-filled
- An initial rise then a fall, or failure of the CVP to rise by 3 cmH$_2$O, implies the circulation is empty and more fluid should be given.

Central venous oxygen saturation ($ScvO_2$) measurement

- If cardiac output is low in relation to tissue oxygen demand, more oxygen will be extracted per unit of blood and the saturation of venous blood will fall
- A true mixed venous oxygen sample taken from the pulmonary artery reflects the balance between tissue oxygen delivery and consumption, a surrogate estimate can be obtained from the SVC (NB right atrial and IVC samples are not reliable)
- Normal $ScvO_2$ is approximately 80%
- Values <70% imply that cardiac output is low and, if there is other evidence of tissue hypoperfusion, there may be benefit in acting to increase cardiac output (e.g. with fluids and inotropes)
- If the $ScvO_2$ is >70%, there is probably little value in increasing cardiac output further with inotropes.

Intra-aortic balloon counter pulsation (aortic balloon pump)

Intra-aortic balloon pump (IABP) devices are mostly used in specialist cardiac units but are increasingly used in emergency departments and intensive care. Indications and contraindications are in the box opposite.

How they work

- A long (34 or 40 cm) balloon is placed in the proximal descending aorta. Rapid expansion of the balloon in diastole displaces blood and promotes flow distally to the mesenteric, renal, and lower limb vessels
- Augmented flow also occurs proximal to the balloon, to the head and neck vessels and coronary arteries
- Flow in coronary vessels mainly occurs in diastole and use of an IABP is associated with a substantial improvement in coronary perfusion
- Abrupt balloon deflation at the start of systole decreases the afterload resistance to left ventricular contraction, improving performance and decreasing cardiac work
- The balloon is inflated and deflated with helium via a pressurized line, fed from a reservoir cylinder
- Inflation and deflation cycles are timed from the surface ECG and adjusted so that the balloon inflates immediately after aortic valve closure and deflates at the end of diastole.

Practical considerations

Insertion and maintenance of IABP devices is a specialist skill and beyond the scope of this text. The following points may be of value in managing patients under your care:

- Most patients receive systemic anticoagulation with IV heparin
- IABP therapy is less effective in patients with tachycardia, especially if the rhythm is irregular. These patients may need specialist review with inflation/deflation cycles being triggered by changes in aortic pressure rather than the surface ECG
- In the event of IABP failure (balloon rupture, exhausted helium supply, ECG trigger failure) pumping must be resumed in 10–15 minutes or the balloon catheter removed. A static IABP is a potential source of clot formation and distal arterial embolization
- IABP catheters can be inserted directly or via a sheath into the femoral artery. At the time of removal, the used balloon will not however retract through the sheath. The IABP catheter should be slowly withdrawn until the balloon reaches the sheath. At this point resistance will be encountered. The sheath and balloon catheter are then pulled out together as a single unit. Pressure haemostasis will be required as for any arterial line (NB: IABP devices tend to be 8F or bigger and prolonged compression will be required)
- Some patients require weaning from IABP support. The usual method is to reduce the balloon inflation frequency to every second, and later to every third cardiac cycle
- Though it is possible to draw arterial blood samples from the pressure monitoring line of an IABP, this should be avoided as the calibre of the line is narrow and prone to blockage if contaminated with blood.

Intra-aortic balloon pump insertion

Indications
- Cardiogenic shock
- Intractable myocardial ischaemia
- Severe pulmonary oedema
- Severe mitral regurgitation with cardiac failure
- Ventricular septal defect with severe cardiac failure (esp. post-MI)
- Support during CABG and coronary angioplasty.

Contraindications
- Significant aortic regurgitation
- Significant aortic stenosis
- Hypertrophic obstructive cardiomyopathy with significant gradient
- Significant peripheral vascular disease (relative contraindication).

Cautions
- May worsen renal and mesenteric blood flow
- ⚙ Peripheral vascular compromise can occur, usually affecting the leg on the side of insertion, though ischaemia of the contralateral limb can also occur. A cold, pale and painful limb with reduced pulses demands immediate specialist attention.

Chest pain

Diagnosing chest pain *16*
Patterns of presentation *16*
Causes of chest pain *17*
Associated physical signs *18*
Investigations *19*

Diagnosing chest pain

- *Nature* of the pain: what is its quality, distribution and severity?
- *Associated features:* e.g. diaphoresis (sweating), breathlessness, (pre)syncope, cough, sputum/haemoptysis, or superficial tenderness
- *Pattern* of occurrence: exacerbating and relieving factors—relationship to exertion, emotional stress, eating, and respiration
- *Change* in frequency or intensity of chest pain
- History of cardiac, respiratory, or upper gastrointestinal pathology?
- Medication, cardiac risk factors, smoking history.

Patterns of presentation

① **Angina pectoris** (📖 p.46) is typically 'tight', 'heavy' or 'compressing' in quality with retrosternal location ± radiation to (left) arm or throat and occasionally to the back or epigastrium. The severity is highly variable from barely perceptible to frightening.

- Chronic stable angina is provoked by physical exertion, cold (leading to peripheral vasoconstriction), and emotional stress and is relieved by rest. Sublingual glyceryl trinitrate, where truly effective, will work within a couple of minutes
- Unstable angina (📖 p.62) occurs at rest or on minimal exertion and is more likely to be severe and sustained. There may be associated 'autonomic features' such as sweating and nausea ± vomiting. There may have been a period of stuttering or rapidly increasing symptoms leading up to the acute presentation. Sharp stabbing pains, pains that are well localized e.g. left submammary, of fleeting duration e.g. <30 seconds or of flitting location are unlikely to reflect myocardial ischaemia.

▶ Remember that angina does not necessarily indicate coronary artery disease. Aortic stenosis, left ventricular outflow tract obstruction, and anaemia are possible causes of angina too.

:⚙: **Thoracic aortic dissection** (📖 p.169) typically has abrupt, even instantaneous, onset. A tearing sensation from anterior to posterior in the chest may be described. The pain is severe and often terrifying. Other features may supervene, according to compromised vascular territories e.g. angina, neurological symptoms due to carotid or spinal artery involvement. The usual cause is hypertension, which may be previously undiagnosed. Marfan syndrome is an important predisposition.

① **Pulmonary embolism** (📖 p.190) may present with pleuritic chest pain (sharp, localized pain, intensified by inspiration). There may be associated breathlessness or haemoptysis. Large pulmonary emboli may diminish cardiac output to the extent that syncope occurs. Ask about risk factors such as prolonged immobility (travel, surgery—especially orthopaedic), malignancy, post-partum, previous DVT/PE, personal or familial tendency to thrombosis, smoking and oral contraceptive use.

⑦ **Pericarditis** (📖 p.182) may also cause pleuritic pain. The pain is often relieved by leaning forward, most likely by easing the apposition of the inflamed pericardial layers. There may be associated 'viral-type' symptoms or features of the underlying disease. Breathlessness may indicate the accumulation of pericardial fluid, even tamponade (📖 p.184).

⑦ **Oesophageal pain** can mimic angina to the extent that it may be associated with physical exertion and may be relieved by nitrates. Association with acid reflux, exacerbation when supine, with food or alcohol and relief from antacids points towards oesophageal pain, but the distinction can be difficult and investigation is often required. Remember that meals can also provoke angina.

Causes of chest pain

Cardiovascular

- Angina/MI 📖 p.46
- Pulmonary embolus 📖 p.190
- Aortic dissection 📖 p.170
- Pericarditis 📖 p.182
- Myocarditis 📖 p.79.

Non-cardiovascular

- Pneumonia
- Pneumothorax
- Chest wall pain (pleuritic/musculoskeletal)
- Muscular
- Oesophageal reflux
- Oesophageal rupture
- Nerve root pain
- Herpes zoster.

Associated physical signs

Unstable angina and acute MI (📖 p.46) Note pulse (either tachycardia or bradycardia occur) and blood pressure. Pay attention for any signs of heart failure. Since things can change quickly it is important to document normal and negative findings clearly, so that new problems will be immediately apparent. Record the heart sounds including any added sounds and the nature or absence of murmurs. A rapid survey for neurological deficits is appropriate (as anticoagulation or thrombolysis may be indicated) with more detailed examination reserved for those where relevant abnormalities are identified.

Pulmonary embolism (📖 p.190) Sinus tachycardia, hypotension, cyanosis, tachypnoea, low grade fever, palpable right ventricle, loud pulmonary component of second heart sound (loud P2), pleural rub, signs of deep vein thrombosis.

Pericarditis (📖 p.182) Pericardial friction rub. Check the pulse character, measure the blood pressure yourself (pulsus paradoxus if systolic pressure difference through respiratory cycle >10 mmHg). Look for other signs of tamponade e.g. hypotension, Kussmaul's sign (JVP rises on inspiration) and quiet or absent heart sounds.

Investigations

Investigations will reflect the possible diagnoses and complications based on the history and physical examination. They will also be directed towards risk factors and secondary prevention measures e.g. cholesterol measurement and treatment in ischaemic heart disease. More detailed consideration of the investigation and management is given on the chapters that deal with each condition.

Unstable angina/acute MI (📖 p.46)

- FBC and U&E
- Glucose
- Total cholesterol and HDL cholesterol
- Troponin
- ECG
- Chest X-ray
- *Selected patients:* echocardiogram, coronary angiography.

Pulmonary embolism (📖 p.190)

- FBC
- D-dimer
- Arterial blood gases
- ECG
- Chest X-ray
- *Selected patients:* CT pulmonary angiogram, ventilation perfusion (VQ) scan, echocardiogram, pulmonary angiogram, Doppler ultrasound leg veins, thrombophilia screen.

Aortic dissection (📖 p.170)

- FBC and U&E
- Group and save blood → cross match
- ECG
- Chest X-ray
- Contrast CT thoracic and abdominal aorta
- *Selected patients:* Transthoracic and/or transoesophageal echocardiogram, MRI.

Pericarditis (📖 p.182)

- FBC and U&E
- CRP
- Troponin
- ECG
- *In selected patients:* ANA, dsDNA, viral titres, pericardial fluid microscopy and culture, echocardiogram.

Shortness of breath

Diagnosing breathlessness 22
Causes of breathlessness 23
Investigations 24

Diagnosing breathlessness

▶ Ask about speed of onset, associated symptoms, previous cardiac and respiratory history, current medication, allergies, cardiac risk factors, smoking history. Obtain additional information from relatives, GP, notes.

▶ Read the ambulance sheet—it is a vital source of information.

Speed of onset

• Sudden	—PE, arrhythmia, acute valve disease, pneumothorax, airway obstruction
• Minutes	—angina/MI, pulmonary oedema, asthma
• Hours/days	—pneumonia, exacerbation of COPD, congestive cardiac failure, pleural effusion
• Weeks/months	—constrictive/restrictive cardiomyopathy, pulmonary fibrosis, pneumonitis
• Intermittent	—asthma, left ventricular failure, arrhythmias.

Associated symptoms

• Chest pain	—ischaemic (angina, MI)
	—pericarditic (pericarditis)
	—pleuritic (pneumonia, PE)
	—musculoskeletal (chest wall pain)
• Palpitation	—AF is the commonest clinical arrhythmia
• Wheeze	—asthma/COPD
• Orthopnoea, paroxysmal nocturnal dyspnoea	
	—cardiac failure
• Sweats/weight loss	—malignancy, infection
• Cough/sputum	—pneumonia
• Haemoptysis	—PE, pink froth suggests pulmonary oedema
• Hyper-anxious	—thyrotoxicosis, anxiety. Breathless that *only* occurs at rest is unlikely to be pathological.

Associated signs

• Clammy, pale	—left ventricular failure, MI
• Cardiac murmur	—valve disease—but beware incidental murmur
• Crackles	—early/coarse—pulmonary oedema, pneumonia
	—late/fine—fibrosis
• Clubbing	—malignancy, cyanotic congenital heart disease
	—endocarditis
• Cyanosis	—severe hypoxaemia
• Displaced apex	—left ventricular dilatation
• RV heave	—elevated right heart pressures
• Elevated JVP	—right heart failure, fluid overload
	—pericardial tamponade/constriction
	—large PE
• Stridor	—upper airway obstruction
• Peripheral oedema	—right heart failure
• CO_2 retention flap	—hypoventilation.

Causes of breathlessness

Cardiovascular
- Left ventricular failure ± pulmonary oedema 📖 p.68
- Angina/MI 📖 p.46
- Severe ± acute ± decompensated valve disease 📖 p.88
- Arrhythmias (especially AF) 📖 p.140
- Constrictive pericarditis/cardiac tamponade 📖 p.186
- Restrictive cardiomyopathy 📖 p.82
- Pulmonary embolus 📖 p.190
- Pulmonary hypertension 📖 p.196.

Non-cardiovascular
- Pneumonia
- Asthma
- Chronic obstructive pulmonary disease
- Pneumothorax
- Pleural effusion
- Upper airway obstruction
- Pneumonitis/pulmonary fibrosis
- Anaemia
- Thyrotoxicosis
- Metabolic e.g. acidosis
- Chest wall pain (pleuritic/musculoskeletal)
- Skeletal abnormalities
- Neuromuscular (diaphragmatic weakness)
- Anxiety/psychogenic.

Respiratory failure
- Diagnosed if the PaO_2 <8 kPa
- Subdivided according to the $PaCO_2$:
  - **Type 1:** $PaCO_2$ < 6.5 kPa. Seen in virtually all acute disease of the lung e.g. pulmonary oedema, pneumonia, asthma
  - **Type 2:** $PaCO_2$ > 6.5 kPa. The problem is hypoventilation. Neuromuscular disorders, severe pneumonia, drug overdose, COPD.

Investigations

- ECG (ischaemic changes, arrhythmias)
- Chest X-ray
- Arterial blood gases
- FBC (anaemia, white cell count)
- Cardiac enzymes (troponin, creatine kinase)
- Further investigations according to differential diagnosis:
  - B-type natriuretic peptide (if low then cardiac failure unlikely)
  - D-dimers (unlikely PE if negative)
  - CRP
  - Blood cultures if pyrexial
  - Peak expiratory flow rate
  - Echocardiography (left ventricular function, valve disease).

Syncope

Introduction *28*
Diagnosing syncope *28*
Causes *29*
Investigations *30*
Neurally-mediated (vasovagal) syncope *32*
Orthostatic hypotension *32*
Cardiac syncope *34*

Introduction

*'A transient, self-limited sudden loss of consciousness, usually
leading to falling'*

Syncope can be caused by a wide spectrum of conditions, ranging from
the benign faint to potentially fatal cardiac arrhythmias. The challenge is
to identify those that require specialist management.

- 1 in 4 of the population will have at least one episode of syncope
- The underlying mechanism is hypotension due to a failure of cardiac
  output or a loss of peripheral vascular resistance. This results in reduced
  cerebral perfusion and consciousness is lost
- Loss of cerebral blood flow of 6–8 seconds may be all that is required
  for syncope to occur
- Syncope can occur without warning but in some, there are prodromal
  symptoms such as nausea, sweating, loss of balance or altered vision
- Patients with true syncope do not remember hitting the ground.

Diagnosing syncope

- The history and examination are the most important steps in
  differentiating between syncopal and non-syncopal causes
- Conditions that mimic syncope include epilepsy, hypoglycaemia, and
  intoxication
- Remember that many elderly patients with syncope describe the
  episodes as falls, often failing to recognize loss of consciousness
- Some conditions without a real loss of consciousness may mimic syncope
  (falls, cataplexy, psychogenic syncope, transient ischaemic attacks).

Questions to ask

- Enquire about the 3 'P's:
  - *Provocative* factors (fatigue, dehydration, warm atmospheres,
    emotional circumstances, fear, pain)
  - *Prodromes* (nausea, sweating, giddiness, abdominal discomfort)
  - *Postural* components (standing, sitting or lying)
- Try to obtain a witness account of the episode. Ask about the
  appearance of the patient during the episode. Was there pallor? Was
  there seizure activity and if so for how long? Remember that short
  lived seizures and myoclonic jerks often occur in simple vasovagal
  syncope
- How long did the episode last? Arrhythmic syncope can be very brief
  with almost immediate recovery such as intermittent atrioventricular
  block (Stokes–Adams attacks). Vasovagal episodes tend to be a little
  longer although these too can be quite short lived
- How long did the patient take to recover and how did they feel? Was
  there confusion? Following vasovagal episodes patients may report
  nausea/vomiting and prolonged light headedness with recurrent
  syncope or presyncope if they stand too quickly. They may also feel
  profound tiredness which can last for hours and often patients report
  sleeping in the immediate aftermath of episodes.

Causes

Neurally-mediated syncope and orthostatic hypotension are the cause of over 50% of cases of syncope. Cardiac causes represent 15% of cases. Neurological and psychiatric causes are found in 10%.

Neurally-mediated (reflex) syncope

- Vasovagal syncope
  - Classical (simple faints)
  - Non-classical (unprovoked)
- Situational syncope
  - Swallow, cough, micturition
- Carotid sinus hypersensitivity.

Orthostatic hypotension

- Autonomic failure
  - Primary (e.g. pure autonomic failure, multi-system atrophy and Parkinson plus syndromes)
  - Secondary (diabetes mellitus)
- Drug induced (vasodilator therapy)
- Volume depletion (diuretics, fluid loss and Addison's disease).

Cardiac arrhythmia

- Sinus node dysfunction (📖 p.128)
- Atrioventricular block (📖 p.132)
- Paroxysmal arrhythmias (📖 p.136)
- Inherited syndromes e.g. long QT, Brugada syndrome (📖 p.34)
- Drug induced bradycardia or prolonged QT interval (📖 p.160).

Other cardiovascular

- Obstructive valvular disease (e.g. aortic stenosis 📖 p.112)
- LV outflow obstruction (e.g. hypertrophic cardiomyopathy 📖 p.80)
- Aortic dissection (📖 p.170)
- Pericardial tamponade (📖 p.184)
- Pulmonary hypertension (📖 p.196)
- Pulmonary embolus (📖 p.190)
- Atrial myxoma (📖 p.282).

Investigations

- 12-lead ECG. Abnormalities suggesting a cardiac cause include:
  - Q waves (prior MI)
  - LBBB or RBBB and left anterior or posterior hemiblock
  - Atrioventricular block (2° or higher) 📖 p.132
  - Sinus bradycardia (<50bpm) or sinus pauses >3 seconds
  - Pre-excitation (short PR interval and delta wave) 📖 p.152
  - Prolonged QT interval 📖 p.160
  - Widened QRS (>0.12s)
  - RBBB with ST elevation in V1–V3 (Brugada syndrome) 📖 p.34
- CXR—cardiac enlargement or aortic dissection (📖 p.170)
- Routine blood testing has a low yield
- Carotid sinus massage
- *In selected patients*: echo, 24 hour tape (see below), tilt table testing.

Who needs a 24 hour ECG tape?

Prolonged ECG monitoring is available in most hospitals. However the diagnostic yield is low in unselected patients with syncope, and will be most beneficial in those with frequent symptoms or in whom you have a high suspicion of a cardiac cause. Factors which suggest a cardiac cause include a history of cardiac disease, an abnormal ECG (see above) or abnormal echo.

Who should be admitted?

Most patients who present following a single episode of syncope can be investigated as an out-patient. In-hospital monitoring and investigation is warranted if the initial clinical evaluation suggests significant structural heart disease or when syncope is recurrent or disabling.

Patients without clinical evidence of structural heart disease and no family history of sudden death who present with an isolated episode of classical vasovagal or situational syncope can be discharged back to their GP without the need for any specific follow-up. All other patients should be referred on for further evaluation.

riving and lifestyle restrictions

⚠ Documented advice on driving **must** be given to each patient presenting with syncope. Restrictions for driving should be reviewed according to national guidelines as updates are made frequently.

Weblink
- In the United Kingdom, the Driver and Vehicle Licensing Agency issue guidelines for medical practitioners http://www.dvla.gov.uk/at_a_glance/content

Other lifestyle restrictions
Patients should be advised to avoid situations where syncope would be hazardous e.g. working up a ladder.

⊙ Neurally-mediated (vasovagal) syncope

- Loss of consciousness in vasovagal syncope is typically for less than 30 seconds although patients and relatives usually report longer
- Likely in the absence of cardiac disease and if there are provoking factors, associated prodromal autonomic symptoms or syncope occurs with head rotation (carotid sinus pressure)
- Situational syncope occurs when directly linked with swallowing, micturition or coughing.

Investigations
- Carotid sinus massage
- Tilt-table testing.

If tests are negative and symptoms recur then consider prolonged ECG monitoring or an implantable loop recorder.

Management

Carotid sinus syndrome (see opposite) usually responds well to dual chamber permanent pacing.

For other neurally-mediated syncope, treatment is less straight forward and patients should be referred for specialist advice.

- Non-pharmacological measures are the first line treatments for patients with vasovagal syncope. These include education, reassurance, tilt-training (enforced upright posture), leg crossing or hand grips during prodromes (to delay or avoid loss of consciousness)
- Pacing for vasovagal syncope can reduce symptoms in selected patients but patients must be informed that it does not prevent attacks
- Pharmacological agents have an unpredictable response and include betablockers, fludrocortisone, midodrine and fluoxetine.

⊙ Orthostatic hypotension

Commonly occurs after standing up or after prolonged standing, typically in a hot crowded room. Can occur after exertion. A systolic blood pressure drop of >20 mmHg after 3 minutes of standing or a drop to <90 mmHg is defined as orthostatic hypotension, irrespective of whether symptoms occur.

The commonest cause is vasodilator drugs and diuretic therapy, especially in the elderly.

rotid sinus massage

Used to diagnose carotid sinus hypersensitivity
Perform with continuous ECG recording and (ideally) beat-to-beat
blood pressure monitoring since blood pressure changes are rapid
- With the patient supine, pressure is applied to each carotid sinus in
  turn for 5–10 seconds. If no abnormal response is elicited, the
  procedure can be repeated with the patient tilted upright
- Avoid in patients with a history of recent stroke (<3 months),
  carotid bruits or known carotid vascular disease.

Carotid sinus hypersensitivity is defined as a ventricular pause of over
3 seconds or a drop in systolic pressure of over 50 mmHg.

Carotid sinus syndrome is the combination of syncope and carotid sinus
hypersensitivity, in a patient in whom clinical evaluation and investigation has identified no other cause of syncope.

Tilt-table testing

- A provocation test for neurally-mediated syncope
- There are a number of protocols in use in clinical practice varying
  in the angle of tilt (typically 60–70 degrees head-up), the duration
  of tilt (20–45 minutes) and the use of additional provocation
  (sublingual GTN)
- Both false positives and false negatives can occur but the test
  compares favourably with other non-invasive cardiac investigations
- Tilt testing is very likely to be positive in those with obvious classical
  vasovagal episodes
- However, the diagnosis is rarely in doubt in such patients and tilt
  testing has a much more important role in investigating patients with
  recurrent unexplained syncopal episodes and in the investigation
  of patients with a broad range of disturbances of consciousness
  where the cause is unclear (i.e. is it really epilepsy?).

Cardiac syncope

- Likely in the presence of severe structural heart disease, particularly severe left ventricular impairment
- Syncope in patients with poor cardiac function confers a bad prognosis
- Symptoms can occur at any time
- May be provoked by exertion
- Can occur whilst sitting or supine
- Can be associated with palpitation or chest discomfort.

Investigations
- Echocardiography
- Prolonged ECG monitoring
- *In selected patients*: Electrophysiological studies
- Syncope occurring during effort should be investigated with echocardiography and exercise stress testing.

Important causes of cardiac syncope
▶ Urgent cardiology referral is required.

Severe left ventricular impairment (📖 p.82)
Associated with monomorphic VT, atrial arrhythmias, postural or drug-induced hypotension.

Aortic stenosis (📖 p.112)
Exertional syncope resulting from severe aortic stenosis is associated with a high incidence of sudden death.

Hypertrophic cardiomyopathy (📖 p.80)
Syncope occurs in up to 25% of patients and can be a risk marker for sudden cardiac death.

Long QT syndrome (📖 p.160, *ECG* 📖 p.339)
Episodes of polymorphic VT can result in recurrent syncope.

Brugada syndrome (*ECG* 📖 p.340)
A cause of sudden cardiac death. ST elevation is seen in the right precordial leads (V1–V3) but changes can be dynamic.

References

European Society of Cardiology guidelines on the management, diagnosis and treatment of syncope. (2004). *Europace* **6**, 67–537.

Palpitation

Introduction *38*
Diagnosing palpitation *38*
Investigations *40*
General management *40*

Introduction

Symptom of increased awareness of the heartbeat

The term however is interpreted by patients to mean different things and it is important to elicit exactly what the patient's symptoms are.

Diagnosing palpitation

The history is vital. A good history can often provide the diagnosis and may avoid the need for further investigation, especially if a non-cardiac cause is suspected. ECG documentation of the cardiac rhythm during an episode is proof of the diagnosis—if this is normal, an arrhythmic cause for the symptoms is excluded.

In general, if the symptoms are brief (<10 seconds), not associated with other severe symptoms and/or occur only at times of stress/anxiety, it is unlikely there is a concerning cause for them.

1. Clarify the symptoms—ask the patient to 'tap out' the rhythm

- Pounding heart — —may be physiological
- Sudden one-off 'jump' — —unimportant, likely ectopic beat
- Irregular heart beat — —likely multiple ectopic beats or AF
- Fast heart rhythm — —consider tachyarrhythmia.

2. What is the pattern? — Likely cause(s)

- Abrupt onset/cessation — SVT, VT, AF
- Slow increase/decrease — Sinus tachycardia
- At times of stress/anxiety — Anxiety/emotion
- Related to exertion — Sinus, AF, SVT if abrupt onset
- Early beat, pause then heavy beat — Ventricular ectopic beats
- Irregular rhythm — AF, multiple ectopic beats.

3. What is the frequency?

- Useful for determining impact on patient
- Guides choice of investigation.

4. Duration of symptoms — Likely cause(s)

- Brief (few seconds) — Atrial/ventricular ectopics
- Several minutes/few hours — SVT/AF
- Continuous — Sinus tachycardia/thyrotoxicosis.

5. Associated symptoms (warrant further cardiac investigation)

- Angina
- Syncope or near syncope
- Significant breathlessness.

6. Previous history

- Known poor LV function — —VT more likely
- Previous SVT/AF/VT — —recurrence?

₁uses of palpitation

₁ardiac

- Tachyarrhythmia:
  - Atrial fibrillation 📖 p.140
  - Atrial flutter 📖 p.144
  - Supraventricular tachycardia (SVT) 📖 p.150
  - Ventricular tachycardia 📖 p.156
- Ventricular or atrial ectopic beats.

Non-cardiac

- Sinus tachycardia—pain, anxiety, fear, exertion, hypoxia, infection, hypovolaemia (e.g. dehydration), anaemia, thyrotoxicosis
- Thyrotoxicosis—appropriate referral to endocrine team. Consider beta-blockade (propanolol 40 mg qds po) ± carbimazole (40 mg daily po) if severe (HR >140 bpm)
- Gastro-oesophageal reflux
- Anxiety/emotion
- Rare:
  - Phaeochromocytoma
  - Carcinoid syndrome.

Investigations

- *12-lead ECG*—ideally during symptoms
- *Blood tests*
  - FBC—anaemia → sinus tachycardia?
  - Thyroid function—thyrotoxicosis?
  - U&E—low/high K^+? (encourages arrhythmias).

Assuming that by this stage, you think a true arrhythmia may be present, further investigations may be undertaken:

- *Echocardiogram*
- *Ambulatory ECG monitoring*—ECG documentation of an arrhythmia prior to management is crucial—treatment is only appropriate when you know what you're dealing with! Assuming this has not been obtained previously, it is worth considering ambulatory monitoring to attempt to document the rhythm during a symptomatic episode. It is worth persevering until an ECG is recorded during symptoms
  - 24/48 hour ECG monitor: good for frequent symptoms, may need several before rhythm identified
  - Patient activated event recorder. The ECG, stored during an episode, can be downloaded to ECG department over the telephone. Device may be kept for several weeks ∴ good for less frequent episodes. Patient needs to be alert during episode and capable of operating device
  - Implantable loop recorders—a small device implanted under the skin in pectoral or axillary region. It typically records 40 minutes of ECG, 'frozen' by a patient-activated key or stored automatically. Good for infrequent but severely symptomatic events.

General management

- Establish rhythm and treat accordingly (see box for relevant sections)
- Most investigations are best performed on an outpatient basis
- Admit if significant associated symptoms for further investigation and ECG monitoring:
  - Severe chest pain
  - Severe SOB
  - Syncope/near syncope.

Specific conditions

Acute coronary syndromes

Acute coronary syndromes (ACS) 46
Pathophysiology 46
Acute ST elevation myocardial infarction 48
Reperfusion therapy 52
Complications of acute MI 58
Unstable angina and non ST elevation MI 62

Acute coronary syndromes (ACS)

Comprise acute ST segment elevation MI (STEMI), non ST segment elevat
MI (NSTEMI) and unstable angina (an ACS without elevation of tropor.
or cardiac enzymes).

Pathophysiology

Understanding the pathophysiology helps to explain the spectrum of
presentation and underpins rational treatment.

Chronic stable angina occurs when fixed stenotic lesions impede myocardial perfusion at times of increased oxygen demand.

Acute coronary syndromes, in contrast, occur when erosion or rupture of
the 'fibrous cap' overlying an atherosclerotic lesion exposes intensely
thrombogenic material within the plaque to platelets and coagulation
factors in the blood. Such lesions need not be stenotic prior to the acute
presentation, which explains why many ACS events are unheralded. The
nature of the occlusion (partial or total; transient, intermittent or fixed)
and location (proximal or distal and the specific coronary artery affected)
largely determine the clinical presentation and course.

Risk factors for coronary atherothrombosis

• Tobacco smoking
• Family history
• Diabetes mellitus
• Hypertension
• Elevated low density lipoprotein-cholesterol (LDL)
• Low level of high density lipoprotein-cholesterol (HDL).

Additional risk factors

• Elevated markers of inflammation, including C-reactive protein,
  interleukin-6 and tumour necrosis factor
• Central obesity
• Sedentary lifestyle
• High apolipoprotein B (ApoB)
• Low apolipoprotein AI (ApoAI)
• High lipoprotein (a) [Lp(a)]
• High plasma homocysteine.

Non-atherosclerotic causes of acute MI

These warrant consideration in specific patients but are less common.
• Embolus e.g. vegetation in infective endocarditis
• Spontaneous coronary dissection
• Intense spasm e.g. in cocaine abuse
• Coronary arteritis (e.g. Kawasaki disease)
• Thrombosis *in situ* in pro-coaguable states
• Trauma—avulsed coronary artery
• Aortic dissection
• Iatrogenic due to coronary intervention.

...sification of acute coronary syndromes

	Troponin	ECG
..EMI	↑ or ↑↑	ST elevation Left bundle branch block
Non-STEMI	↑ (occasionally ↑↑)	Normal Abnormal, but unchanged ST segment depression T wave inversion
Unstable angina	↔	

:Ọ: Acute ST elevation myocardial infarction

This is a medical emergency usually caused by thrombotic occlusion o major epicardial coronary artery. Irreversible ischaemic injury to th myocardium is threatened (or may have occurred at presentation) Prompt action conserves myocardium and prevents complications, including death.

Symptoms

- Severe 'crushing' central chest pain ± radiation to jaw, neck or arms
- 'Autonomic' features: diaphoresis (sweating), nausea and vomiting
- Breathlessness due to left ventricular dysfunction
- Atypical presentations include pain in the back or abdomen, confusion
- MI may be silent (especially in the elderly and in patients with diabetes).

Determine

- Timing of the onset of symptoms
- Are there contra-indications to thrombolysis? (p.55)
- Has aspirin been given e.g. in ambulance?
- Is there a history of coronary disease?

Signs

- Pain or distress
- Clammy (sweating and cutaneous vasoconstriction) and grey.

Look for complications
- Hypotension
- Lung crepitations and other evidence of heart failure
- Rhythm disturbances (bradycardia e.g. heart block; AF, sinus tachycardia (pain, anxiety or compensatory)
- Murmurs (mitral regurgitation due to papillary muscle ischaemia or chordal rupture; acquired ventricular septal defect (p.59)
- Fever <38°C is common in the first 48 hours.

Investigations

12-lead ECG

If ST segment elevation is present, a rapid decision on reperfusion ther-apy is required. See indications (p.53).
- In patients with inferior MI, right sided ECG leads should be obtained, to identify possible right ventricular infarction
- Where ECG-diagnostic criteria are not met initially, but pain persists, obtain serial ECGs every 10 minutes
- A portable chest radiograph should be obtained but, where the clinical diagnosis is acute MI, CXR should not delay reperfusion therapy
- Blood for troponin, and repeated 12 hours after symptom onset. In acute MI, initial treatment decisions are NOT dependent on blood test results
- FBC, U&E, serum cholesterol and glucose. Remember that serum cholesterol may decrease after 24 hours and persist at lower level for several weeks after acute MI.

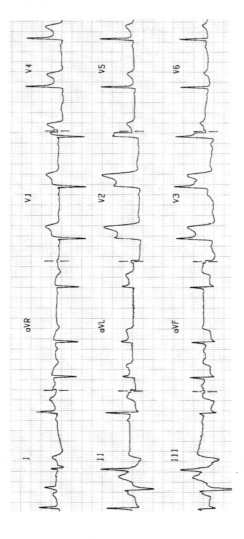

ECG in acute anterolateral MI. There is marked ST segment elevation in leads V1–V4 and aVL. Reciprocal ST segment depression is present in leads II, III and aVF.

Coronary artery anatomy

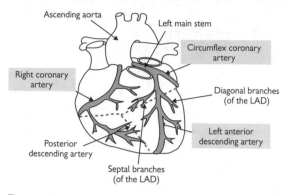

There are three principal coronary arteries. The **left main stem** arises from the left aortic sinus and soon gives rise to the **(1) left anterior descending** and **(2) circumflex** coronary arteries. The **(3) right coronary** artery has a separate origin in the right aortic sinus.

The **left anterior descending** (LAD) coronary artery runs in the anterior interventricular groove supplying the *anterior wall* of the heart. It gives off **septal** branches that supply blood to the *anterior 2/3 of the interventricular septum*, including the *left bundle branch*; **diagonal** vessels to the *lateral wall* of the left ventricle and has a terminal bifurcation that supplies the *apex* of the left ventricle and sometimes wraps around to supply the *inferior wall* of the left ventricle.

The **circumflex** (LCX) artery runs posteriorly in the left atrioventricular groove giving **obtuse marginal** branches to the *lateral wall* of the left ventricle and supplying the *posterior wall* of the left ventricle.

The **right** coronary artery (RCA) runs in the right atrioventricular groove. It gives branches to the *sino atrial node, atrioventricular node* and *right ventricle*. On reaching the posterior interventricular groove, it gives rise to the **posterior descending artery** that supplies the *inferior wall* of the left ventricle, and the *inferior 1/3 of the interventricular septum*. This is the more common variant. In about 10% of patients, the circumflex gives rise to the posterior descending artery and is then termed 'dominant'.

...s of arterial occlusion	Myocardial territory	ECG changes
...AD	Antero-lateral	V_4–V_6; I, VL
	Antero-septal	V_1–V_4
		LBBB
LCX	Posterior	Mirror image changes in V_1–V_2 or V_3 i.e. ST segment depression ± inferior changes; tall R in V_1
		May be electrically silent on standard 12-lead ECG
RCA	Inferior wall of LV	II, III, aVF
	Right ventricle	ST elevation V_4R to V_6R

Interpreting the troponin measurement

Troponins are contractile proteins, specific to the myocardium, and elevated levels in the blood are indicative of myocardial injury. Levels rise within 12 hours of myocardial injury, peak at around 24 hours and remain elevated for up to 14 days.

It is important to recognize that the diagnosis of acute coronary syndrome is, in the first instance, clinical—the initial management is based on clinical diagnosis and the ECG(s) and is not contingent on the troponin result. The troponin may turn out to be elevated and in NSTEMI patients is one of the markers of increased risk (📖 p.65) but importantly, may be normal in patients with unstable angina who are at high risk of subsequent cardiac events, and the clinical diagnosis is crucial in these patients.

Furthermore, release of troponin T is not specific to coronary disease. Caution is necessary in interpreting an elevated serum troponin in the absence of a typical history and/or ECG changes, particularly where the rise is relatively modest. Other conditions that can lead to troponin elevation include:

• Myocarditis
• Pericarditis
• Pulmonary embolism
• Sepsis
• Renal failure.

Because of superior specificity, troponin measurement has largely superceded measurement of creatine kinase, AST and LDH.

▶▶ **Immediate management**
- Oxygen
- Aspirin 150–300 mg chewed for rapid buccal absorption
- IV access
- Diamorphine 2.5–5 mg IV or morphine 5–10 mg IV
- Metoclopramide 10 mg IV
- Oral beta blocker e.g. atenolol 50 mg po or metoprolol 25–50 mg tds in the absence of heart failure and hypotension (BP <100 mmHg). Intravenous beta blockers e.g. atenolol 5–10 mg IV can also be used particularly to counter tachyarrhythmias or marked hypertension
- Clopidogrel 75–300 mg po
- ▶ *Reperfusion therapy*: Primary PCI or thrombolysis (see below).

▶ Your patient may be terrified. Provide reassurance where possible.

☼ **Reperfusion therapy**

Make sure that you are familiar with the acute MI protocol of your institution. Most hospitals have multi-disciplinary teams (e.g. CCU nurse-led) to accelerate provision of reperfusion therapy. The goals are prompt restoration of coronary flow and myocardial perfusion. Delays increase myocardial necrosis, decrease the efficacy of eventual reperfusion therapy and increase mortality. Reperfusion therapy with thrombolysis or with percutaneous coronary intervention (PCI) is acceptable. Rapid action is vital: the door-to-needle time (thrombolysis) should be <20 minutes and the door-to-balloon time (for primary PCI) should be <60 minutes.

Primary percutaneous coronary intervention

Primary PCI refers to immediate PCI as the initial reperfusion strategy. It achieves high levels of vessel patency and, in experienced hands, may reduce mortality compared to thrombolysis. The risk of stroke is also lower compared to thrombolysis.
- Initiate immediate management measures (see above)
- Alert the cardiac catheterization laboratory/duty cardiologist at the earliest opportunity. Ideally the patient is moved from the Emergency Department (or ambulance) directly to the cardiac catheterization laboratory.
- In discussion with the interventional cardiologist, it is reasonable to start the glycoprotein IIb/IIIa receptor inhibitor abciximab once the decision for primary PCI has been made
- Informed consent is usually obtained by the operator or a competent deputy
- If there is likely to be more than minor delay (i.e. >60 minutes door-to-balloon) before PCI, thrombolysis may be more appropriate, particularly if the symptom duration is less than 3 hours.

...ations for reperfusion therapy

- ...mptoms of myocardial ischaemia
- ...Onset within the prior 12 hours (or up to 24 hours if symptoms of ...ischaemia persist)
- ...ST segment elevation of >0.1 mV (usually 1 mm) in at least two adjacent limb leads
- or ST segment elevation of >0.2 mV (usually 2 mm) in at least two contiguous chest leads
- or new (or presumed new) left bundle branch block
- or true posterior MI*.

*Posterior MI is notorious for the absence of definitive ECG changes. ST segment depression in leads V2 and V3, particularly in the context of concomitant inferior and/or lateral ST segment elevation, should suggest posterior MI, where the clinical syndrome fits.

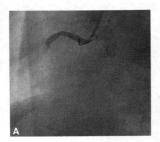
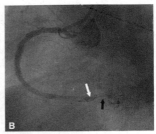
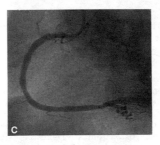

(A) Acute myocardial infarction with occlusion of the right coronary artery. A small filter device (B, arrows) captures embolic debris released during primary percutaneous intervention. Stent deployment at the site of occlusion restores vessel patency and distal flow (C).

Thrombolysis

Practical considerations mean that for many hospitals thrombolysis the standard reperfusion treatment. Even then, primary PCI should considered in patients with contraindications to thrombolysis or th <75 yrs old with shock and within 36 hours of an acute MI.

- Exclude contraindications (opposite) and warn of the small risk of stroke (~0.5%)
- Avoid arterial punctures, multiple venous punctures and intramuscular injections in patients where thrombolysis is likely.

Choice of thrombolytic

Both streptokinase and alteplase (rt-PA) reduce mortality. Alteplase results in 10 fewer deaths per 1000 patients treated, at the expense of 3 additional strokes compared to streptokinase. Angiographic patency and flow at 90 minutes in the infarct-related artery are directly related to 30-day mortality. Even with rt-PA, the patency is only 80% at 90 minutes. The single bolus agent tenecteplase (500–600 micrograms per kilogram [max 50mg]) has equivalent efficacy to accelerated tPA. Reteplase (10 units over not more than 2 minutes followed by 10 units 30 minutes later) has similar efficacy.

- rt-PA accelerated regimen (<6h from symptom onset):
  - If >65 kg body weight (weight-adjust dose if <65 kg)
  - 15 mg by iv bolus followed by
  - 50 mg over 30 minutes, then
  - 35 mg over 60 minutes (i.e. total 100 mg over 90 min)
- Treatment with rt-PA should be followed by a bolus and infusion of intravenous unfractionated heparin (trials on the use of low molecular weight heparin in this setting are ongoing).

Alternatively:

- Streptokinase 1.5 million units over 60 minutes
- Tenecteplase (TNK) 500–600 micrograms per kilogram (max 50 mg) over 10 seconds.

Reperfusion is suggested by resolution of ST segment elevation by >50% following thrombolysis and relief of pain.

Failure to reperfuse

Failure of symptoms and/or ST segment elevation to resolve by >50% 60–90 minutes after thrombolysis may result from a failure to achieve patency of the epicardial vessel or due to distal (microvascular) occlusion. The optimal course of action is uncertain. There is no clear benefit from repeat thrombolysis or from 'salvage/rescue' PCI. Trials to resolve this uncertainty are ongoing. Salvage PCI is usually recommended in the presence of ongoing symptoms or electrical or haemodynamic instability.

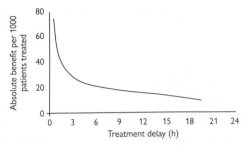

Summary of meta-analysis of thrombolysis trials shows the marked time sensitivity of thrombolysis particularly within the first 'golden' two hours after the onset of pain. Modified from Boersma E, Maas AC, Deckers JW et al. (1996). *Lancet* **348**, 771–775.

Contraindications to thrombolysis

Absolute
- Any prior intracranial haemorrhage
- Known intracranial structural vascular lesions (e.g. arteriovenous malformation)
- Known intracranial malignant neoplasm (primary or secondary)
- Ischaemic stroke within 3 months
- Active bleeding or bleeding diathesis
- Significant head trauma within 3 months.

Relative
- Severe hypertension (systolic >180 mmHg; diastolic >110 mmHg) despite treatment
- Traumatic or prolonged CPR
- Major surgery within 3 weeks
- Non-compressible vascular punctures
- Recent (within 2–4 weeks) internal bleeding
- Pregnancy
- Active peptic ulcer
- Current anticoagulant use
- Pain for >24 hours
- For streptokinase: prior exposure to streptokinase (persistent antibodies).

▶ NB: Patients with contraindications to thrombolysis should be considered for primary PCI.

Modified from Antman EM, Anbe DT, Armstrong PW *et al.* (2004). ACC/AHA guidelines for the management of patients with ST elevation myocardial infarction. *Circulation* **110**, 588–636.

Additional treatments

- An ACE inhibitor e.g. ramipril 2.5 mg od or lisinopril 5 mg od should be commenced within the first 24 hours following acute MI if the systolic blood pressure is >100 mmHg. There is particular benefit in the presence of left ventricular dysfunction. The dose should be titrated upwards as blood pressure permits
- Statin treatment should be instigated in almost all patients
- The anti-platelet agent clopidogrel administered at presentation and continued at a dose of 75 mg daily for 4 weeks, in addition to standard therapy, reduces the 30-day risk of a composite of death, re-infarction and stroke inpatients undergoing non-invasive management
- In post STEMI patients with left ventricular ejection fraction <40%, already receiving an ACE inhibitor and with either symptomatic heart failure or diabetes, but without significant renal dysfunction or hyperkalaemia, there is a benefit from aldosterone blockade
- Diabetic patients should receive an insulin infusion based on a sliding scale.

Risk stratification and prognosis

An important predictor of 30-day mortality in acute MI is the presence (and degree) of heart failure, quantified by Killip in 1967 and updated from GUSTO trial data for the thrombolytic era (📖 p.57).

The extent of myocardial damage can be estimated from the magnitude of the rise in cardiac enzymes/troponin and from the appearances on echocardiography.

Important differential diagnoses

☼ *Aortic dissection* (📖 p.170) can present with chest pain and ST segment elevation. The pain is usually distinguished by its abrupt onset, migration to the back and tearing nature. Where ST segment elevation is recorded, it is usually in the inferior (i.e. right coronary) territory since dissection involving the left main stem is usually fatal.

❶ Thrombolytic therapy in acute aortic dissection is potentially lethal. Where there is significant suspicion of dissection, further imaging (e.g. contrast CT aorta, transoesophageal echo or MRI) should be obtained.

⑦ *Acute pericarditis* (📖 p.182) may present with chest pain and ST segment elevation on the ECG. The pain is typically exacerbated by inspiration and relieved by sitting upright. The ECG changes are classically concave upwards (saddle shaped) and may be widespread, spanning the equivalent of multiple coronary territories.

MI, prognostic indicators

p	Clinical feature	30-day mortality(%)
p class I	No S3 and clear lungs	5.1
...lip class II	S3 or crepitations in lungs	13.6
Killip class III	Crepitations >50% of lung	32.2
Killip class IV	Shock	57.8
Anterior MI		9.9
Inferior MI		5.0
Age <60y		2.4
Age 60–75y		7.9
Age >75y		20.5

Adapted from Lee KL, Woodlief LH, Topol E J et.al. (1996). Predictors of 30-day mortality in the era of reperfusion for acute myocardial infarction. Circulation 91, 1659–1668.

Complications of acute MI

Immediate complications (*within hours*)

Ventricular arrhythmia

Ventricular tachycardia and ventricular fibrillation are the principal cau~~se~~ of death early in acute MI. Patients in the immediate peri-infarct perio~~d~~ should be managed on a specialized coronary care unit that is equipped to treat such arrhythmias (📖 p.154,156).

Complete heart block (CHB)

Usually occurring in the context of acute inferior MI, CHB is often transient, resolving with reperfusion. Where haemodynamic compromise occurs, insertion of a temporary transvenous pacing wire may be indicated. Resolution of CHB may take several days, so be patient before prescribing a permanent pacemaker. Complete heart block in the context of anterior MI suggests extensive infarction, and adverse prognosis. Temporary pacing should be considered (📖 p.296).

Hypotension

Hypotension in the absence of signs of heart failure may respond to a fluid challenge e.g. 250–500 mL normal saline given rapidly. Acute inferior MI is often accompanied by right ventricular infarction.

① Right ventricular infarction

Occurs in 30% of inferior MI. Suggested by ST elevation >1 mm in V_4R. Carries an adverse prognosis. Often associated with hypotension, which may require robust fluid resuscitation to maintain left-sided filling pressures.

Cardiogenic shock (📖 p.4).

Where hypotension (systolic BP <90 mmHg) is accompanied by signs of heart failure or where left ventricular function is known to be severely impaired, intravenous fluid challenge is contra-indicated. It may be appropriate to institute inotropic support (📖 p.8) and/or intra-aortic balloon counter pulsation (📖 p.12). Within 36 hours of acute MI, emergency PCI should be considered.

Pulmonary congestion and pulmonary oedema

Give oxygen, morphine, and intravenous loop diuretics e.g. furosemide 40–100 mg IV. Infuse GTN 0.5–10 mg/hour IV if BP >90 mmHg systolic. Obtain a CXR. Insert a urinary catheter and monitor urine output hourly. Give oxygen and monitor HbO_2 saturation with pulse oximetry. In severe cases, CPAP or intubation and ventilation may be required (📖 p.10). Anticipate these requirements and discuss early with the ITU physicians. Speak to the patient's relatives.

complications (*within days*)

einfarction

prisingly, the optimal course of action in reinfarction following initially ccessful reperfusion is uncertain. Many would proceed to angiography nd PCI (or coronary artery bypass) in the presence of ongoing symp- oms or electrical or haemodynamic instability. It is reasonable to re-administer thrombolysis in patients for whom PCI is not available within 60 minutes (NB streptokinase should not be given more than once).

▶▶ *New murmur* and abrupt haemodynamic deterioration suggest the possibility of papillary muscle rupture (or dysfunction), ventricular septal defect or free wall rupture. Obtain an echocardiogram urgently. In general a structural problem needs a structural fix. Call the surgeons early.

☼: Mitral regurgitation (MR)

Acute severe MR due to papillary muscle rupture is a cardiac surgical emergency. Stabilization can be attempted with intravenous diuretics, intravenous nitrates, and intra-aortic balloon counterpulsation (📖 p.12) but these are temporizing measures at best. Urgent surgical repair should be considered.

☼: Ventricular septal rupture

Acquired VSD requires urgent surgical repair. Stabilization can be attempted with intravenous diuretics, intravenous nitrates, and intra-aortic balloon pump insertion (📖 p.12).

☼: Rupture of myocardial free wall

Abrupt deterioration within 3 days post MI may indicate myocardial rupture. If not fatal, urgent surgical repair should be considered.

⑦ Pericarditis

Common after myocardial infarction. The pain is usually pleuritic, positional and distinct from the ischaemia-related pain of the initial presentation. Pericarditis occurs >12 hours after acute MI and is treated with high (anti-inflammatory) dose aspirin, up to 650 mg 4–6 hourly. There is some evidence that indomethacin and ibuprofen may adversely affect myocardial remodeling early post-MI. Anticoagulation should be stopped if a pericardial effusion develops or enlarges.

Mural thrombus and systemic embolization

Full anti-coagulation with heparin (and subsequently warfarin) should be obtained in patients with large anterior MI, known LV thrombus or atrial fibrillation all of which are associated with an increased risk of systemic embolization. Aspirin should usually be continued.

Late complications (*several weeks*)

⑦ *Dressler syndrome*

Auto-immune mediated acute febrile illness that occurs 2 weeks to sev~~e~~ months after acute MI. The incidence has fallen in the reperfusion e~~ra~~ Management is with aspirin or NSAIDs. Large pericardial effusions ma~~y~~ accumulate causing haemodynamic embarrassment or even tamponade. Obtain an echocardiogram. Stop anti-coagulants to minimize risk of haemorrhagic transformation. Percutaneous drainage may be required (📖 p.300).

Ventricular tachycardia

Scar formation post myocardial infarction predisposes to ventricular tachycardia (📖 p.156). In selected patient implantable cardioverter-defibrillator (ICD) therapy is indicated.

Left ventricular aneurysm

Infarcted tissue may become thinned and dyskinetic. Aneurysms are haemodynamically inefficient, predispose to thrombus formation and may cause persistent ST elevation on the ECG.

Post infarct management

In the absence of complications or persistent ischaemia, patients should be mobile within 24 hours. At day 5–7, a pre-discharge submaximal exercise test may be undertaken. A low-level positive test indicates further myocardium at risk, and pre-discharge angiography is usually indicated. A negative test indicates a low-risk group and is helpful to rebuild patient confidence.

Inform the patient that they may not drive for one month and of their responsibility to inform the licensing authority and their motor insurance company.

Take the opportunity to implement education on secondary prevention e.g. smoking cessation and diet (low saturated fat, low salt, promote Mediterranean-type diet). Introduction to a supervised, structured rehabilitation programme is generally beneficial.

Discharge medication

- Aspirin
- Beta-blocker
- ACE inhibitor
- Statin
- Clopidogrel.

Weblinks

American Heart Association/American College of Cardiologists joint guidelines on management of acute ST segment elevation MI. (2004). *Circulation* **110**, 588–636.
http://circ.ahajournals.org/cgi/reprint/110/9/e82

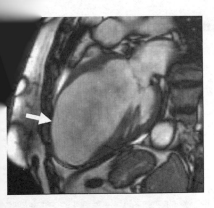

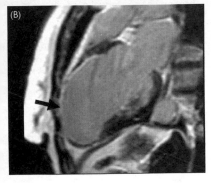

(A) Cardiac MRI following acute anterior and apical myocardial infarction. Note thinning of the LV anterior wall and apex (white arrow). Blood within the heart appears white. (B) Late enhancement imaging with gadolinium shows the full extent of the infarcted tissue (infarcted myocardium appears white, black arrow).

① Unstable angina and non ST elevation MI

In the absence of sustained ST segment elevation, ischaemic pain abruptly worsening severity or occurring at rest is classed as 'unstable angina' or non ST segment elevation MI (NSTEMI). The distinction depends on the eventual presence (NSTEMI) or absence (UA) of an elevated troponin measurement. The underlying pathology (ruptured or eroded coronary plaque with non-occlusive or intermittently occlusive thrombus) and initial management is the same. The immediate objectives are to relieve pain and to prevent progression to acute MI.

Symptoms

Central chest pain of various severity and duration, possibly radiating to the jaw or (left) arm and typically not relieved by glyceryl trinitrate. Pain is sometimes accompanied by 'autonomic' features diaphoresis (sweating), nausea and vomiting. There may be a history of prior chronic stable angina.

Signs

Pain or distress, clammy (a result of sweating and cutaneous vasoconstriction). Occasionally accompanied by intermittent pulmonary oedema, depending on degree of ischaemia and underlying left ventricular function. There may be no abnormal physical signs.

Investigations

At presentation, the diagnosis is clinical.
- The ECG may be normal
- ECG changes include ST segment depression and T wave inversion, which may be 'dynamic'—coming and going with symptoms
- Exclude sustained ST segment elevation (📖 p.48)
- If the ECG is normal but pain persists, obtain serial ECGs
- Check FBC (to exclude anaemia)
- Troponin at presentation and 12 hours after onset of pain.

▶ Immediate management

- Oxygen
- Aspirin 150–300 mg chewed to achieve rapid buccal absorption
- Clopidogrel 300 mg po then 75 mg daily
- Low molecular weight heparin
- Sublingual or intravenous glyceryl trinitrate
- Morphine 5–10 mg or diamorphine 5–10 mg IV analgesia
- Metoclopramide 10 mg IV
- Beta-blocker e.g. atenolol 50 mg po or metoprolol 25–50 mg po tds
- Oral diltiazem is an alternative when beta-blockers are contraindicated (and there is no evidence of cardiac failure, atrioventricular block or hypotension)
- ± Revascularization in selected patients according to risk.

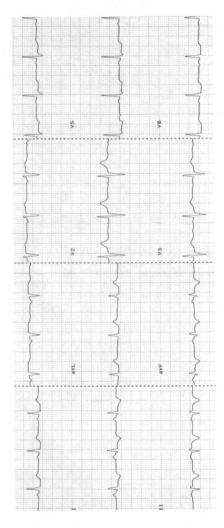

ECG during chest pain. ST segment depression in leads I, V5 and V6 with T wave inversion in leads II, III and aVF is suggestive of ischaemia in the inferolateral territory.

Glycoprotein IIb/IIIa inhibition

Glycoprotein IIb/IIIa inhibitors are potent anti-platelet agents that block the common path of platelet aggregation. Patients undergoing PCI may benefit from administration of abciximab prior to the procedure, while patients with 'high risk features' (see below) or evidence of ongoing or ischaemia may benefit from eptifibatide or tirofiban (but not abciximab) even where early PCI is not planned.

Risk stratification and early invasive treatment

Evidence from randomized trials suggests that higher risk patients derive greatest benefit from a strategy of early coronary angiography and revascularization (PCI/coronary artery bypass).

Clinical indications for early invasive strategy include ongoing symptomatic ischaemia (especially dynamic ST segment depression on the ECG), haemodynamic compromise, and recent (e.g. within 6 months) PCI. Elevated troponin also suggests a high risk category. The TIMI score is a well-validated, simple risk calculator (see box). As a guide, patients with TIMI score >3 are at high risk and early invasive management may be beneficial.

Recent percutaneous coronary intervention

Insertion of a metallic stent during PCI poses a risk of acute and subacute stent thrombosis. To counter this, the anti-platelet agents aspirin and clopidogrel should be given prior to PCI. Heparin (± abciximab) is given in the cardiac catheterization laboratory. The risk of stent thrombosis declines rapidly during first 24 hours after PCI. For conventional bare metal stents, it is usual to continue a combination of aspirin 75 mg od and clopidogrel 75 mg od for at least one month after PCI to cover the small risk of subacute stent occlusion. Where drug-eluting stents are used, there is a possibility of delayed stent endothelialization and aspirin/clopidogrel combination is usually maintained for 6 months.

① Be aware of the possibility of stent-related thrombosis, particularly early after implantation, where drug compliance is questionable or where anti-platelet agents have recently been stopped. Early angiography is indicated.

TIMI Risk score for unstable angina/NSTEMI (1 point or each)

- Age ≥ 65 years
- ≥ 3 coronary risk factors
- Use of aspirin within 7 days
- Elevated cardiac markers
- ST segment deviation
- Prior angiographic evidence of coronary disease
- More than 2 angina events within 24 hours.

The score is determined by simply summing the number of risk factors above. For patients with TIMI score 0–1, the combined risk of death, (re)infarction or recurrent severe ischaemia requiring revascularization is about 5% while TIMI score 6–7 confers a risk of 41%.

Weblinks

American Heart Association/American College of Cardiologists joint guidelines on management of unstable angina and NSTEMI. (2002). *Circulation* **106**, 1893–1900.
http://circ.ahajournals.org/cgi/content/full/106/14/1893

Acute heart failure

Introduction 68
Clinical features 68
Management 70
Monitoring and goals 74
Special circumstances 76
Cardiogenic shock 78
Myocarditis 79
Cardiomyopathies 80
Difficult case examples 84

Introduction

Acute heart failure can be either acute or acute-on-chronic (more common). In all cases, efforts should be made to identify the underlying cause, and in particular, why it should present now. Heart failure is not a homogeneous condition and whilst some general principles apply, successful treatment depends upon the accurate assessment of the aetiology and haemodynamic profile in each patient.

Clinical features

Clinical features are of fluid overload and low cardiac output:

Fluid overload/congestion
- Orthopnoea
- Raised JVP*
- Gallop rhythm
- Pulmonary inspiratory crackles
- Peripheral oedema*
- Ascites*
- Hepatic distension*.

Low output
- Tachycardia
- Low blood pressure/narrow pulse pressure*
- Cool extremities
- Poor capillary refill
- Confusion/drowsiness
- Oliguria
- Pulsus alternans (terminal).

* May be absent in acute heart failure.

:©: If patient is shocked (systolic BP <90 mmHg with signs of reduced major organ perfusion), they need urgent attention (🕮 p.6).

Causes of decompensation

Many cases of acute heart failure are in fact decompensation of chronic heart failure, and $^2/_3$ are a readmission within 3 months. Seeking the reasons for decompensation are therefore important. Failure to comply with therapy (either drugs or fluid intake) is a common cause.
- Lack of compliance
- Uncontrolled hypertension
- Arrhythmias
- Inadequate therapy
- Pulmonary infection
- Administration of inappropriate medications (e.g. NSAIDs, antiarrhythmic agents, non-dihydropyridine calcium antagonists)
- Fluid overload (often iatrogenic if in hospital)
- Myocardial infarction
- Endocrine disorders (thyrotoxicosis).

Investigation
- FBC (anaemia, infection)
- U&E
- Troponin (acute coronary syndrome)
- Thyroid function
- ECG (ischaemia, MI)
- Brain natriuretic peptide (BNP)—see box
- Echocardiography
- Arterial blood gas analysis if severe heart failure.

...ology of acute heart failure

- ...chaemic heart disease
- Valvular heart disease
- Arrhythmias
- Hypertension (either longstanding, or crisis)
- Pericardial tamponade
- Myocarditis
- Cardiomyopathy with acute decompensation (dilated, hypertrophic, post partum)
- Aortic dissection (coronary ischaemia, aortic regurgitation)
- Renal failure (volume overload)
- Alcohol abuse
- High output (anaemia, hyperthyroidism, arteriovenous fistulae).

Brain natriuretic peptide (BNP)

Serum levels are now recommended to confirm the diagnosis of acute heart failure. BNP is more accurate than any other single finding on history, examination or laboratory testing. A negative test result makes the diagnosis of heart failure unlikely. Threshold values of >300 pg/mL for NT-proBNP and 100 pg/mL for BNP have been suggested. The availability of diagnostic testing may however be limited.

The following may give rise to an elevated BNP in the absence of clinical heart failure:
- Renal failure
- Acute coronary syndromes
- Aortic stenosis
- Mitral regurgitation
- Hypertrophic cardiomyopathy.

Systolic vs. diastolic heart failure

Systolic heart failure is characterised by reduced systolic function on echocardiography or other imaging modality. Diastolic heart failure is characterised by abnormalities of left ventricular filling in the absence of major systolic dysfunction. This is mainly due to increased stiffness of the ventricle, commonly from longstanding hypertension. These patients respond to vasodilators, adequate fluid balance and rate slowing (if tachycardic); they respond poorly to dehydration. Diastolic heart failure is particularly common in the elderly.

Differential diagnosis

Any cause of SOB (📖 p.22) may be included here, but the comm ones, particularly without CXR evidence of pulmonary oedema, are:

- Chronic obstructive pulmonary disease.
- Pulmonary embolus (major pulmonary embolism can however cause pulmonary oedema).

Echocardiography is the most useful diagnostic tool for discrimination and may be supplemented by BNP measurement (see above).

For patients presenting with radiological evidence of pulmonary oedema, non-cardiogenic causes have to be considered (see box). Clinical features suggestive of a non-cardiogenic cause are normal/low venous pressure, normal/increased cardiac output, normal ECG, normal LV function on echo, failure to respond to standard heart failure therapy.

Management

Immediate management

Treatment aims are to reduce preload and afterload with a combination of diuretics and vasodilators. It is important in the early stages of treatment to establish adequate oxygenation—this has a major impact on myocardial performance and the response to diuretic therapy.

- Oxygen therapy
- IV morphine 2.5–10 mg IV (good venodilator and relieves acute stress)
- Loop diuretics (e.g. furosemide 40–120 mg IV)
- IV nitrates (e.g. GTN 1–10 mg/hr) may be useful if significant failure and BP allows (i.e. >95 mmHg systolic)
- Withdraw any drugs which may be contributing to heart failure (e.g. calcium channel blockers and NSAIDs).

Continuing management

Drug therapy can be tailored according to the haemodynamic profile of tissue perfusion and fluid overload (see opposite).

ACE inhibitors

- Not usually introduced in the acute phase of heart failure although there is evidence for their early introduction in patients following MI
- In the long term, they are beneficial, including a reduction in mortality
- They should be withdrawn temporarily in the following circumstances:
  - Systolic BP <80 mmHg or <100 mmHg in the presence of renal impairment or diuretic resistance
  - Creatinine >300 mmol/L
  - Progressive rise in creatinine of >25–30%
- They can be introduced/reintroduced when fluid status is optimal and the patient is haemodynamically stable.

Beta-blockers

- Contraindicated in acute heart failure
- In all but mild cases with predominant fluid overload, they should be withdrawn temporarily
- Can be (re)introduced when the patient has been stabilised, and fluid balance is optimal—may be weeks later.

Causes of non-cardiogenic pulmonary oedema

- Imbalance of Starling's forces
  - Increased pulmonary capillary pressure
  - Decreased plasma oncotic pressure (hypoalbuminaemia)
  - Decreased interstitial pressure (decompression of pneumothorax, severe asthma)
- Increased alveolar-capillary permeability (ARDS)
  - Infection
  - Toxins
  - Aspiration of gastric contents
  - Disseminated intravascular coagulation (DIC)
  - Acute pancreatitis
- Drugs
- 'Shock-lung'
- Other
  - Lymphatic insufficiency
  - High altitude
  - Pulmonary embolism
  - Neurogenic
  - Eclampsia
  - Post CABG/cardioversion
  - Post anaesthesia.

Haemodynamic profiles in heart failure

(warm/cold = peripheral perfusion; wet/dry = congested/not congested)

Warm and wet (common)
- Emphasis on diuretic therapy with addition of vasodilators
- Significant diuresis may be required
- Beta-blockers can be continued
- Inotropes inappropriate.

Cold and wet
- Emphasis on vasodilator therapy with additional diuretics
- Beta-blockers and ACE inhibitors may need temporary withdrawal
- Vasodilating inotropes (e.g. dobutamine) may be helpful if poor response.

Warm and dry
- Target profile
- Emphasis on titration of chronic therapy to optimal doses.

Cold and dry
- ▶ Distinguish from hypovolaemic shock
- Emphasis on inotropic support ± intra-aortic balloon pump
- Haemodynamic monitoring required
- Cautious filling if CXR clear.

From Nohria A, Lewis E, Stevenson LW. (2002). Medical management of advanced heart failure. *JAMA* **287**, 628–640.

Diuretics

Loop
- Standard therapy in acute pulmonary oedema and in patients demonstrating signs of fluid overload
- Infusions are more effective than bolus regimens (time above the natriuretic threshold is more important than maximum concentration in the nephron)
- Start with furosemide 40 mg IV/bumetanide 1 mg IV if not on diuretics or, if previously treated, with normal oral dose given intravenously and titrate according to response
- In severe heart failure, diuretic resistance or renal impairment consider furosemide bolus followed by infusion over 4–8 hours. Maximum bolus dose 100 mg, maximum infusion rate 4 mg/min.

Non-loop
- Thiazides and aldosterone antagonists are useful as an adjunct to loop diuretics in diuretic resistance
  - Bendroflumethiazide 2.5 mg daily/hydrochlorthiazide 25–50 mg twice daily (ineffective when the creatinine clearance is <30 mL/min)
  - Metolazone (2.5–10 mg daily) has an effect regardless of creatinine clearance and produces a more rapid diuresis. Care is required however due to its potent effect
- Aldosterone antagonists
  - Spironolactone (25–50 mg daily), eplerenone (25–50 mg daily). Avoid if creatinine >220 umol/L or K^+ >5mmol/L.

Digoxin
- If fast AF and acute heart failure, often beneficial
- For those in sinus rhythm, opinion is divided as to the usefulness in acute settings. It is most effective in patients with a 3rd heart sound, elevated JVP and severe left ventricular dilatation.

Vasodilators
- Morphine (2.5–10 mg IV stat)
  - Predominant venodilator
  - Important in relieving acute distress
- Nitrates
  - IV if acutely unwell (e.g. GTN 1–10 mg/hr)
  - Oral may be added, though evidence for usefulness is poor
  - Venodilators at low doses; arterial vasodilators in high dose
  - Tolerance occurs after 24 hours
  - Aim for a 10 mmHg fall in systolic blood pressure
  - Discontinue if blood pressure falls below 90 mmHg
- Sodium nitroprusside (0.5–5 µg/kg/min IV infusion) 📖 p.174
  - For severe cases
  - Requires arterial pressure monitoring
  - Prolonged use is associated with toxicity and should be avoided in patients with severe renal or hepatic failure
  - Most useful in hypertensive heart failure and acute mitral regurgitation.

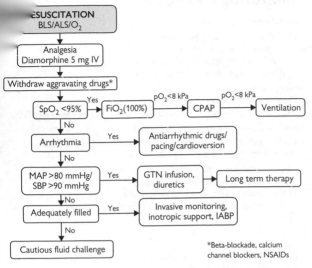

Management algorithm for patients presenting with acute heart failure.

Monitoring and goals

Monitoring

Pulse, BP, ECG monitoring, pulse oximetry
- Automatically in first 24 hours
- Prolonged in the presence of arrhythmias, during inotrope therapy or in the case of persistent haemodynamic instability.

Arterial blood gases
- On admission in all cases with severe heart failure
- Regularly in patients on continuous positive airways pressure (CPAP)

Electrolytes, creatinine and renal function
- Daily in patients who are haemodynamically unstable, and patients on intravenous or combination diuretics.

Fluid balance/urinary catheterization
- Fluid balance recommended in all cases
- Urinary catheterization recommended in severe heart failure and is a useful surrogate for cardiac output in the absence of significant renal disease.

CVP (p.11)
- Not usually required
- Not recommended in acute pulmonary oedema (lying patient flat may precipitate cardiac arrest)
- May be required for inotropic support.

Pulmonary artery catheter (p.294)
- Rarely required
- Useful for exclusion of non-cardiogenic pulmonary oedema
- May be misleading in mitral stenosis, aortic regurgitation, high airway pressures and poor LV compliance.

Goals of therapy

Without haemodynamic monitoring
- Symptomatic improvement
- Oxygenation SaO_2 >95%
- Warm peripheries
- Systolic BP >90 mmHg
- JVP (isolated right heart failure excluded) <5 cm
- Clinical and radiological resolution of pulmonary oedema
- Urine output >0.5 mL/kg/hr.

With haemodynamic monitoring (above included)
- Pulmonary wedge pressure 16–18 mmHg
- Cardiac output >2.5 L/min/m^2
- Systemic vascular resistance 950–1300 dyne-seconds/cm^2.

New York Heart Association (NYHA) classification of heart failure

Class I	Asymptomatic (though with reduced LV function). No limitation of physical activity.
Class II	Mildly symptomatic, with silght limitation of physical activity. Comfortable at rest but ordinary physical activity results in fatigue or dyspnoea.
Class III	Moderately symptomatic, with marked limitation of physical activity. Comfortable at rest but less than ordinary activity results in fatigue or dyspnoea.
Class IV	Severely symptomatic. Unable to carry out any physical activity without dicomfort. Includes dyspnoea/fatigue at rest, with any activity resulting in increased discomfort.

Special circumstances

Intractable pulmonary oedema and hypoxia
(pO_2 <8 kPa, pCO_2 >6.5 kPa, worsening acidosis).

Non-invasive ventilation

Two forms of non-invasive ventilation can be used: CPAP and BiPA, which has additional inspiratory assistance. These may be particular, helpful in patients with reversible ischaemia. BiPAP may however increase cardiac work, and should be used with caution and after specialist advice.

Invasive ventilation

Should be considered in the following circumstances:
• Failure to correct hypoxia (SaO_2 <90%)
• Fatigue associated with acidosis (pH <7.2)
• Failure to tolerate CPAP mask.

Haemofiltration

May occasionally be required in the presence of acute renal failure and volume overload, where the aetiology of the acute heart failure is felt to be reversible.

① Cardiorenal syndrome
Patients who are anuric or oliguric despite loop diuretic therapy may require inotropic support (📖 p.9) and/or haemofiltration.

Acute MI (📖 p.48)
Revascularization using thrombolysis or primary/rescue angioplasty with balloon pump support if available.

Acute ventricular septal defect/mitral valve rupture
• These predominantly mechanical disorders giving rise to pulmonary oedema often respond poorly to conventional therapy.
• Early surgery with balloon pump support prior to surgery is recommended (📖 p.12).

Diabetes
Insulin infusion is recommended in diabetics with acute heart failure.

Thyrotoxicosis
Cautious use of non-selective beta-blockade is recommended (propranolol 0.5 mg IV, or 10 mg orally).

Hypertensive crisis (📖 p.278)
LV function is often normal.

① Severe bronchoconstriction ('cardiac asthma')
• A profound bronchoconstrictor response to pulmonary oedema
• If conventional therapy fails there may be a response to IV aminophylline (250 mg IV bolus over 20 minutes). Caution however— this is associated with an incidence of cardiac arrhythmias.

heart failure

- rticularly seen in the context of RV infarction (usually accompanying inferior MI) and pulmonary embolism
- The diagnosis is suggested by clear lung fields in the context of a raised venous pressure and systemic hypotension
- Early echocardiography is recommended
- Requires fluid supplementation (200 mL saline fluid challenges 🕮 p.11).

Recurrent admissions with 'flash' pulmonary oedema

These patients may have a relatively normal exercise tolerance between attacks, the following should be considered:

- Renal artery stenosis
- Reversible ischaemia
- Tachyarrhythmias.

① Severe aortic stenosis (🕮 p.112)

- Patients with severe aortic stenosis and heart failure are difficult to treat
- Diuretics are the mainstay of therapy as a holding measure
- Vasodilators and inotropes are contraindicated
- The only truly effective treatment is urgent aortic valve replacement—although high risk, the prognosis is dismal without.

Causes of right heart failure

- RV infarction
- Pulmonary embolic disease
- Tamponade
- Chronic pulmonary disease/hypoxia
- Pulmonary hypertension
- Valvular disease
- Congenital heart disease e.g. Ebstein's anomaly, Eisenmenger syndrome
- Right ventricular dysplasia.

:⚙: Cardiogenic shock

In cardiogenic shock with acute heart failure, prognosis is particu[..]
poor and recovery is unlikely unless there is a reversible cause.

Cardiogenic shock is defined by
- Mean arterial pressure <60 mmHg or systolic BP <90 mmHg
- In the presence of:
  - Satisfactory heart rate (60–95 bpm)
  - Adequate filling pressures
  - On 100% oxygen
- With one of the following:
  - Obtunded
  - Poor peripheral perfusion
  - Low urine output
  - Central venous O_2 saturation <70%
  - Lactic acidosis >2.0 mmol/L.

Treatment (see cardiovascular collapse 📖 p.6)

This is only appropriate in patients where there is a potentially reversible cause or as a bridge to revascularization or transplantation. Principally consists of:
- Inotropic support
- Intra aortic balloon pumping
- Mechanical left ventricular assist devices are available in a few centres, again primarily as a bridge to transplantation.

ⓘ Myocarditis

Causes
- Viral (characteristically enterovirus infections e.g. coxsackie)
- Other infective: bacterial, fungal, rickettsial, and spirochaetal
- Cocaine
- Peripartum cardiomyopathy
- Giant cell myocarditis.

Presentation
A wide spectrum from the acute fulminant form, in which the outcome is death or complete recovery, to a chronic form indistinguishable on presentation from a dilated cardiomyopathy.

Clinical features
- Fatigue, breathlessness and chest discomfort
- There may be a fever with a disproportionate tachycardia
- Atrial and ventricular arrhythmias are common.

Investigations
- CXR: heart size may be normal or enlarged
- ECG: ST and T wave abnormalities, may present with regional ST elevation and can be mistaken for acute MI. AV block and conduction defects
- Echocardiography: global or regional wall motion abnormalities
- Viral serology: often sent but rarely useful in guiding therapy
- Troponin: elevated in acute cases
- Myocardial biopsy: again rarely helpful in guiding therapy but may be performed at the time of coronary angiography.

Treatment
- Bed rest, ACE inhibitors, diuretics and inotropes as required
- Arrhythmias treated as for patients with known LV dysfunction. However, patients display an increased sensitivity to digoxin
- Anticoagulation for severe LV dysfunction or LV thrombus
- Cardiac transplantation in selected cases.

Cardiomyopathies

Hypertrophic cardiomyopathy

The identification of patients presenting with hypertrophic cardiomyopathy is important, as vasodilators and inotropes are contraindicated. The most likely emergency presentations are with syncope, arrhythmias or chest pain. Presentation with LV failure is usually secondary to fast AF.

Symptoms
- Syncope
- Chest pain
- Palpitations
- Breathlessness.

Examination
- Can be normal
- Prominent a wave in JVP
- Bifid pulse and/or apex
- Mid systolic murmur in aortic region
- 4th heart sound
- Pan systolic murmur at apex (if mitral regurgitation).

Investigations
ECG: Prominent Q waves in inferior/anterior leads, left atrial enlargement, giant T wave inversion (apical variant), pre-excitation (see opposite).

ECHO: LVH (>13 mm), systolic anterior movement of mitral valve, mitral regurgitation, outflow tract gradient, diastolic dysfunction.

Treatment
- Arrhythmias treated according to standard guidelines
- Digoxin is best avoided and verapamil should be used cautiously in patients with an outflow tract gradient
- Early cardioversion for AF is advised in patients who are hypotensive and in pulmonary oedema
- Angina can be treated with beta-blockade
- Adequate filling pressures should be maintained, especially in post-operative patients
- In the presence of an outflow tract gradient, inotropes and nitrates are contraindicated, even in the presence of hypotension.

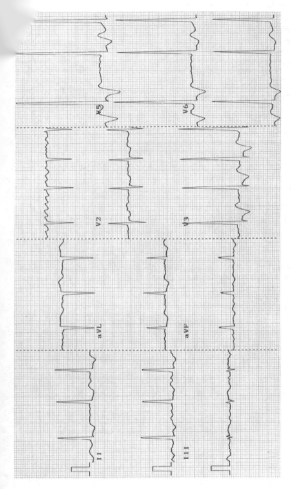

ECG in hypertrophic cardiomyopathy. The underlying rhythm is AF. Tall R waves are seen along with repolarization changes in V3–V6, in keeping with significant LV hypertrophy.

Dilated cardiomyopathy

- Globally dilated LV with poor function
- Treat as for other causes of heart failure
- Causes (see below) and reasons for decompensation should be investigated
- Causes:
  - Idiopathic (± familial)
  - Coronary artery disease
  - Alcoholic cardiomyopathy
  - Hypertension (end-stage)
  - Aortic stenosis (end-stage)
  - Myocarditis
  - Chronic tachyarrhythmia
  - Peri-partum cardiomyopathy
  - Autoimmune disease
  - HIV cardiomyopathy
  - Arrhythmogenic right ventricular cardiomyopathy (predominantly RV dilation, but can be LV too)
  - Haemochromatosis.

Restrictive cardiomyopathy

- Usually hypertrophied LV with poor function (especially diastolic)
- Like hypertensive heart failure, requires adequate filling and vasodilators, and minimal diuretics
- Causes:
  - Idiopathic
  - Myocardial fibrosis (from any cause)
  - Amyloidosis
  - Sarcoidosis
  - Scleroderma
  - Iron storage diseases (haemochromatosis, multiple transfusions in thallassaemia)
  - Diabetic cardiomyopathy
  - Eosinophilic heart disease
  - Glycogen storage diseases
  - Other rare genetic diseases (Fabry's, Hurler's).

Difficult case examples

1. AF and heart failure

Severe pulmonary oedema with AF at a rate of 170. Has not responded to 3 doses of furosemide 40 mg IV stat and a loading dose of digoxin. Oxygen saturations are 90% on 100% O_2. Is it safe to cardiovert?

A: Cardioversion under full anaesthetic is probably the best option here especially if the patient is hypotensive. Cardioversion with sedation alone is not appropriate (due to the significant respiratory compromise already). A period of ventilation afterwards may be needed but this in itself can be a good treatment for heart failure.

2. Sepsis and heart failure

Acute dyspnoea and sepsis, pulse 110 bpm, systolic BP 80 mmHg, venous pressure not visible. There is a history of left ventricular failure and the patient does not want to lie flat. What is the appropriate management?

A: Patients with a combination of sepsis and heart failure present difficult management problems. A clear chest X-ray is reassuring and it is then reasonable to institute fluids, but often there is only a portable X-ray which is difficult to interpret. A central line is helpful with a target CVP of 8–10 mmHg. However, it is not advisable to force a patient flat to put in a central line when they are acutely dyspnoeic: they can arrest. Cautious boluses of 100 mL normal saline can be used but **stay with the patient to monitor the response.** Stop if the patient deteriorates or desaturates. The ITU team should be involved as vasoconstricting inotropes may be needed.

3. Patient on beta-blocker therapy

Presents with breathlessness and evidence of left ventricular failure with basal crepitations and an elevated jugular venous pressure. The patient is taking carvedilol 25 mg bd and an ACE inhibitor. Should the beta-blocker be stopped and if so when can it be restarted?

A: If the patient is haemodynamically stable and is not in acute respiratory distress, it is reasonable to continue beta-blocker therapy and increase the diuretic dose. With haemodynamic compromise (hypotension, systolic BP <100 mmHg or poor perfusion), beta-blocker therapy should be discontinued and restarted when the pulmonary oedema has cleared and systolic blood pressure is ≥100 mmHg. The ACE inhibitor should be stopped if there is severe hypotension (systolic BP <80 mmHg) or moderate hypotension (systolic BP 80–100 mmHg) with evidence of deteriorating renal function (oliguria or rising creatinine).

⋯r peripheral perfusion and pulmonary oedema
⋯ed with pulmonary oedema. The patient is cold peripherally, the
⋯s 100 bpm (small volume) and systolic blood pressure 110 mmHg.
⋯have not passed urine for 2 hours despite 100 mg IV frusemide.
⋯at are the therapeutic options?

Patients with evidence of poor tissue perfusion but a reasonable
systolic pressure may respond to vasodilating inotropes (e.g. dobutamine
or low dose dopamine). Vasodilating inotropes are often started
inappropriately late when the systolic blood pressure is low—in this
situation they are often ineffective and lower the blood pressure further.

5. Cardiogenic shock post-MI

Deteriorated 8 hours following thrombolysis for a large anterior MI.
Pulmonary oedema and hypotension (systolic blood pressure 80 mmHg)
are present. There has been no urine output for 3 hours. What is the
appropriate management?

A: This situation carries a very high mortality regardless of any intervention.
If there is felt to be a significant reversible component then vasoconstricting
inotropes or insertion of an intra-aortic balloon pump is required whilst
awaiting transfer to the catheter laboratory for angioplasty. Advanced
support is not indicated if no definitive procedure to restore myocardial
function is planned.

Valve disease

Acute valve problems 88
Indications for valve surgery 92
Chronic valve disease 94
Infective endocarditis 96
Prosthetic valves 106
Acute rheumatic fever 110
Aortic stenosis 112
Aortic regurgitation 114
Mixed aortic valve disease 114
Mitral stenosis 116
Mitral regurgitation 118
Pulmonary stenosis 120
Pulmonary regurgitation 120
Tricuspid stenosis 122
Tricuspid regurgitation 122

Acute valve problems

Acute valve problems often require urgent treatment, as decompen. heart failure can occur rapidly.

☼ Acute vs. acute-on-chronic vs. cardiac decompensation

It can sometimes be difficult to differentiate the nature of the current problem, as patients' presentation may be similar:

- Acute: Rapid or sudden deterioration of valve function on previously normal (or near-normal) valves. Nearly always regurgitation. The patient is usually extremely unwell as the LV has not had time to compensate
- Acute-on-chronic: Recent worsening of pre-existing valve dysfunction
- Cardiac decompensation: Pre-existing (and unchanged) valve dysfunction but with left and/or right ventricular decompensation.

Causes

☼ *Acute:*

- Infective endocarditis
  - leaflet disintegration, perforation or dehiscence (?abscess)
  - vegetation (→ incompetence or stenosis)
  - dehiscence of prosthetic valve ring
  - papillary muscle rupture
- Myocardial infarction
  - usually mitral regurgitation 2° to papillary muscle dysfunction (causes: papillary muscle infarction, rupture or tethering to infarcted myocardial wall)
- Aortic dissection
  - if type A, can dissect into aortic root and cause aortic valve dehiscence and regurgitation
- Ruptured chordae tendinae
  - mitral, or rarely, tricuspid regurgitation
- Trauma.

① *Acute-on-chronic:*

All the above, plus
- Recent deterioration of valve function as part of the natural history
- Severe changes in haemodynamics (e.g. rise or fall in blood pressure, changes in fluid balance).

① *Cardiac decompensation:*

- Natural history, 2° to chronic valve dysfunction
- Changes in haemodynamics (blood pressure changes or fluid shifts)
- Arrhythmias (particularly tachyarrhythmias)
- Other diseases affecting the myocardium (ischaemic heart disease, hypertensive heart disease, infiltrative diseases etc.).

...ation

..al symptom is *breathlessness*:

...ute valve disease — onset over minutes/hours

...cute-on-chronic — onset over days/weeks (generally)

Cardiac decompensation — onset over hours–months.

Other symptoms may be:
- Angina (aortic stenosis, acute coronary ischaemia)
- Syncope (in aortic or pulmonary stenosis)
- Explosive, tearing back pain in aortic dissection.

Differential diagnosis

▶ It is important to look for other causes of breathlessness (📖 p.23), as even if valve disease is present, it may be an innocent bystander. Previous notes/echocardiograms may be helpful in identifying any recent changes. If no change in valve or LV function has occurred, consider other diagnoses.

Clinical signs
- Signs of significant valve disease (see relevant sections below)
- Signs of cardiac failure
- External stigmata of infective endocarditis
- Absent pulses in aortic dissection.

Investigations

Echocardiography

Any patient with a suspected valvular problem presenting acutely needs an echocardiogram. If you suspect true acute valve dysfunction, emergency echocardiography is required. For presentations over days/weeks (i.e. acute-on-chronic or cardiac decompensation), the echocardiogram can usually wait 24–72 hours, depending on the clinical status of the patient—those who are extremely unwell may need an urgent echo cardiogram. Transoesophageal echocardiography (TOE) may be required for difficult to visualise aortic valves/root, aortic dissection or mitral regurgitation to assess feasibility of mitral valve repair.

Chest X-ray

To confirm pulmonary oedema or look for other causes of SOB.

ECG
- Features of chronic valve disease (LVH—aortic stenosis/regurgitation; broad P wave–mitral stenosis; AF—mitral stenosis/regurgitation)
- Fast AF/other arrhythmia?—cause of acute decompensation?
- Long PR interval—aortic root abscess?
- Acute MI/ischaemia?

Blood tests
- FBC—anaemia causing/exacerbating SOB; high WCC indicating infection (endocarditis, chest, other)
- U&E—reduced renal perfusion, renopathy 2° to endocarditis, high/low K^+ causing arrhythmia, baseline test
- ESR and CRP—infection
- Blood cultures—endocarditis: 3 or 6 sets over 24–48 hrs.

General management
- Identify and treat cause
- Treat heart failure if present—usually diuretics (e.g. furosemide 8⟨ IV or more) ± vasodilators for regurgitant lesions (ACE inhibitors, ⟨ if severe, IV nitrates/sodium nitroprusside 📖 p.70)
- Avoid beta-blockers in aortic regurgitation—these lengthen diastole, and may worsen the AR, and also prevent a compensatory tachycardia.

:☼: Acute valve regurgitation may require urgent transfer to a tertiary centre with cardiothoracic surgical facilities—discuss with cardiologist. These patients are usually very unwell and ITU care may be required. They often need emergency valve replacement surgery.

① For acute-on-chronic lesions and decompensation, most patients need in-patient referral to a cardiologist for consideration of valve replacement surgery. This may be the first presentation with symptoms, which are important for deciding on surgery.

Other, lesion-specific advice is given in the relevant sections of this chapter.

Emergency non-cardiac surgery (see also 📖 p.256)
If a patient needs emergency surgery and has a concomitant valve lesion, this can sometimes present a problem. In practice, regurgitant lesions are rarely a problem—the afterload reduction from anaesthetic agents and hypovolaemia tends to reduce any valve leak.

Severe aortic, pulmonary or mitral stenosis may cause difficulties (moderate disease is rarely a problem). The lack of capacity to increase cardiac output significantly is the major issue, and these patients are at higher operative risk, and require careful attention to fluid balance and haemodynamics—large shifts are to be avoided. In some cases, valve replacement surgery may be required prior to non-cardiac surgery, but the relative risks of valve replacement, delaying the non-cardiac surgery and proceeding with non-cardiac surgery with appropriate care should be assessed. Non-cardiac surgery for a life-threatening condition should clearly proceed, and the increased risk accepted.

Don't forget antibiotic prophylaxis! 📖 p.96.

guide to the commonest murmurs

c stenosis
p.112

- Harsh, rasping, sometimes musical, ejection murmur
- Aortic region, radiating to carotids
- Slow rising pulse, soft/absent A_2, LVH.

Aortic regurgitation
p.114

- Early diastolic, de-crescendo murmur
  (± systolic flow murmur)
- Lower left sternal edge
- Collapsing pulse, displaced, hyperdynamic apex.

OS

Mitral stenosis
p.116

- Low-pitched, quiet, mid-diastolic rumble
- Apex, no radiation
- Opening snap, 'tapping' apex, AF, loud P_2 (pulm HT).

Mitral regurgitation
p.118

- Soft, blowing, monotonous, pansystolic murmur
- Apex, radiating to axilla
- Displaced, hyperdynamic apex.

Grading of systolic murmurs (Levine 1933)
Grade

1 Barely audible
2 Soft but readily detected
3 Prominent
4 Loud, usually with thrill
5 Very loud with thrill
6 So loud, can be heard with the stethoscope just off the chest.

How to recognize an innocent ('flow') murmur

- Soft ejection systolic murmur
- Grade ≤2
- Usually heard along left sternal edge/pulmonary region; occasionally at the apex
- Normal heart sounds
- No associated thrills or added sounds
- No signs of LV dilatation
- Normal ECG and no cardiac abnormalities on CXR.

▶ Innocent murmurs do not need echocardiography.
▶ Diastolic, pan-systolic and loud murmurs (grade 4+) are not 'innocent'.

Indications for valve surgery

☼ Emergency (within few hours)
- Acute valve regurgitation with severe heart failure (NYHA 3 or 4)
- Type A aortic dissection ± aortic regurgitation
- Post-infarct mitral regurgitation
- Ruptured sinus of Valsalva aneurysm.

ⓘ Urgent (in-patient)
- Rapidly increasing SOB or pulmonary oedema with chronic valve lesion
- Unstable prosthetic valve
- Uncontrolled infective endocarditis despite adequate antibiotics:
  - Heart failure due to valve dysfunction
  - Valve obstruction from vegetation/thrombus
  - Fungal and other anti-microbial resistant endocarditis (e.g. Brucella, Coxiella)
  - Cardiac abscess formation (usually aortic root)
  - Persistent bacteraemia (after 7–10 days)[†]
  - Recurrent emboli[†]
  - Large (>10 mm) mobile vegetations (↑ risk of embolization)[†]
- Early prosthetic valve endocarditis (<2 months from implantation).

ⓘ Elective
- Severe aortic stenosis (peak gradient >50 mmHg) with stable symptoms *or* LV dysfunction (EF <50%)
- Severe mitral regurgitation:
  - If symptomatic
  - If asymptomatic with reduced LV function (EF <60%) *or* end-diastolic diameter >7.0 cm *or* end-systolic diameter >4.5 cm
- Severe aortic regurgitation:
  - If symptomatic
  - If asymptomatic with reduced LV function (EF <50%) *or* end-diastolic diameter >7.5 cm *or* end-systolic diameter >5.5 cm
- Moderate–severe valve disease if other cardiac surgery planned.

[†]Relative indication—surgery may be considered.

Chronic valve disease

Most valve lesions are managed conservatively, particularly if patient.
well. In the absence of symptoms or progressive LV dysfunction, ther,
rarely a need for surgery and these patients can be managed in outpa
tients with follow-up, often on an annual basis. Progression to LV dys-
function/excess dilatation or development of symptoms should prompt
consideration of surgery. Mild disease may not need follow up, but does
need prophylaxis against endocarditis (see below).

Antibiotic prophylaxis

Most patients with chronic valve lesions are at risk of endocarditis, and
prophylactic antibiotic therapy should be given before dental and surgical
procedures where there is significant risk (🕮 box p.89).

Useful guidelines

Bonow RO, Carabello B, de Leon C et al. (1998). ACC/AHA guidelines for the management of
patients with valvular heart disease. *Circulation* **98**,1949–1984, and at:
http://circ.ahajournals.org/cgi/content/full/98/18/1949

① Infective endocarditis

This condition still carries a high mortality (15–20%) despite mc
antibiotics. Uncomplicated viridans streptococcal infections may hav
better prognosis, but staphylococcal and prosthetic valve endocardit
carry a high mortality. Potential reasons for the continued high mortality
are: an aging population, ↑incidence of prosthetic endocarditis, ↑lifespan
of patients with congenital heart disease, ↑staphylococcal and fungal
infections, tricuspid valve endocarditis from intravenous drug use, and
antibiotic resistance.

Infective endocarditis is most likely to develop where underlying structural cardiac defects are present, which underlines the importance of
prevention in susceptible individuals. Endocarditis occurring on normal
valves tends to involve the more virulent organisms, especially *Staph.
aureus*. Other factors which increase risk are: ↑susceptibility to infection
(old age, chronic alcoholism, haemodialysis, diabetes, immunosuppres-
sion) and recurrent bacteraemia (inflammatory bowel disease, colon
carcinoma, IV drug use).

Prophylaxis

Prevention of endocarditis is clearly the best option, and antibiotic prophylaxis is recommended for patients at moderate or high risk of endocarditis undergoing certain procedures—see box. Prophylaxis is aimed
mainly at viridans streptococcal and HACEK organisms (📖 p.101), or
Strep. bovis and enterococci for GI/GU procedures.

Other simple measures are equally important in the prevention of bacteraemia, and patients at risk should pay attention to these such as good
oral and feet hygiene and attention to cuts and skin disorders which may
allow bacteria to penetrate the skin (especially in diabetics).

Procedures requiring antibiotic prophylaxis

Dental	Extraction, polishing, scaling, gingival procedures.
GI	Any endoscopic procedure, GI surgery.
GU	Most procedures, except urinary catheterization without infection present.
Respiratory	Bronchoscopy, surgical procedures.
Cardiac	Occlusive device insertion, PPM/ICD insertion & cardiac surgery.

Procedures where antibiotic prophylaxis may be considered

Respiratory	Nasal packing.
Cardiac	Angiography/plasty, TOE.
GU	Smears, vaginal delivery.
Dermatology	Dermatological surgery, burns, acupuncture, tattooing & body piercing.

---

of infective endocarditis

ers to combination of susceptibility to infection and the consequences.

gh risk	• Previous infective endocarditis • Prosthetic heart valves (including bio-prosthetic) • Cyanotic congenital heart disease (e.g. transposition of the great arteries, Fallot's tetralogy) • Surgical systemic-pulmonary shunts.
Moderate risk	• Acquired valvular heart disease (e.g. AS, AR, MR) • Mitral prolapse with regurgitation or severe valve thickening • Non-cyanotic congenital heart disease (e.g. bicuspid aortic valve, primum ASD, PFO, VSD, PDA, coarctation) • Other structural cardiac defects (e.g. aortic root replacement, HCM).

Low risk (does not require antibiotic prophylaxis)

- Mitral prolapse without regurgitation
- Secundum ASD
- Repaired ASD/VSD/PDA (NB percutaneous repair requires prophylaxis for 12 months)
- Post-Mustard or Fontan procedures without residual defect
- Previous CABG
- Permanent pacemaker/ICD
- Innocent heart murmurs.

Antibiotic prophylaxis for patients at moderate & high risk

Standard

Dental, respiratory, or oesophageal procedures in patients *without* prosthetic valves or previous endocarditis.

Normal	**Penicillin-allergic**
Amoxicillin 3 g po 1 hr pre (or 2g IV 30 mins pre).	Clindamycin 600 mg 1 hr pre + 150 mg IV/po @6hrs *or* azithromycin 500 mg po 1 hr pre *or* clarithromycin 500 mg po 1 hr pre *or* vancomycin & gentamicin as below.

Particularly high risk

All procedures for patients with prosthetic valves or previous endocarditis.
All genitourinary & lower GI procedures.

Normal	**Penicillin-allergic**
Amoxicillin 2g IV 1 hr pre +1 g IV/po @6 hrs (& gentamicin 1.5 mg/kg IV 30 mins pre for high risk pts).	Vancomycin 1g IV over 2 hrs, 2 hrs pre (& gentamicin 1.5 mg/kg IV 30 mins pre for high risk pts).

- Patients already on antibiotics should receive an alternative class from the lists above.
- Patients having procedures involving infected tissues should have antibiotic prophylaxis directed at the infection, as this is the most likely source of any endocarditis.

Presentation
May be acute, sub-acute, or occasionally hyper-acute:

- Sub-acute   —insidious onset over months usually
- Acute   —presentation over 1–4 weeks
- Hyper-acute —rapid deterioration over hours/days, usually due to acute valve regurgitation.

While the classical sub-acute presentation, with months of non-specific malaise, still occurs, there is an increasing tendency towards acute presentations, which may reflect increasing numbers of more virulent organisms, e.g. *Staph. aureus* or the HACEK group (📖 p.101).

The presentation is usually with non-specific symptoms and can mimic many other systemic diseases. A high index of suspicion is therefore necessary (see box opposite). Cardiac tumours can sometimes mimic endocarditis (esp. atrial myxoma) and these should also be considered.

Clinical features
These can be divided into four areas, attributable to:

Infection
- Fever
- Night sweats
- General malaise
- Weight loss
- If longstanding: anaemia, clubbing, splenomegaly.

Cardiac involvement
- New/altered murmur
- Signs of severe valve regurgitation
- Left ventricular failure due to valve deterioration or direct involvement of the myocardial endothelium
- Prolonged PR interval if aortic root abscess.

Immunological phenomena
- Microscopic haematuria, glomerulonephritis, generalised vasculitis, arthralgia
- Petechiae, splinter haemorrhages in nail beds, Osler's nodes (tender nodules [infarcts] on finger pulps/palms/soles), Janeway lesions (painless palm/sole erythematous macules)
- Flame/boat-shaped retinal haemorrhages, Roth spots (boat-shaped retinal haemorrhages with pale centre).

▶ Immunological phenomena tend not to occur in acute presentations, as the infection has evolved too quickly for their development. They also do not occur with right-sided lesions.

Emboli
- Commonly: cerebral, retinal, coronary, splenic, mesenteric, renal
- Pulmonary in right-sided endocarditis
- May develop into abscesses, or a mycotic aneurysm.

Potential routes of infection should also be sought (e.g. teeth, skin infections).

...urs and endocarditis

...nuine new murmur in the context of someone who is unwell is ...ly significant and the old adage 'fever + new murmur = endocarditis ...til proven otherwise' is true to an extent. In practice however, knowing ..hether the murmur is new, or a newly-discovered old murmur, can be difficult. However, endocarditis does of course occur commonly on valves with pre-existing lesions (i.e. murmurs) and a change in the character of a pre-existing murmur is suspicious. It should also be remembered that any infection will tend to increase cardiac output and can thus lead to an innocent 'flow' murmur, or a slight change in a pre-existing murmur. Thus, the picture is complicated...!

Therefore, murmurs that are more than 'innocent' (📖 p.93) in the context of non-specific illness require investigation, though by themselves are not diagnostic of endocarditis (see also indications for echocardiography below). In particular, the combination of fever plus murmur (either new or old) is not enough for a diagnosis without other supporting evidence, and antibiotics should NOT be started until other evidence is available, unless the patient is very unwell and a presumptive diagnosis of endocarditis is likely. In all cases, 3 or 6 sets of blood cultures should be taken prior to commencing antibiotic treatment.

Indications for echocardiography in suspected endocarditis
—when level of suspicion is high:
- New valve lesion (usually regurgitant murmur)
- Embolic events of unknown origin
- Sepsis (i.e. bacteraemia plus systemic features) of unknown origin
- Haematuria, glomerulonephritis and suspected renal infarction
- Fever plus:
  - +ve blood cultures for organisms typical for endocarditis
  - High predisposition for endocarditis e.g. prosthetic valve
  - First manifestation of heart failure
  - Newly-developed conduction disturbance or ventricular arrhythmias
  - Typical immunological manifestations of endocarditis
  - Multifocal/rapidly changing pulmonary infiltrates
  - Peripheral abscesses of unknown origin (e.g. renal, splenic, spinal)
  - Predisposition plus recent diagnostic/therapeutic intervention known to result in significant bacteraemia.

NB: *a fever without other evidence for endocarditis is not an indication for echocardiography.*

Diagnosis

The cornerstone of diagnosis is microbiological evidence of in[...]. Although helpful, echocardiography (even TOE) does not exclude [...] docarditis, and can produce false positive results. It is therefore c[...] that an accurate clinical picture is obtained (also to exclude o[...] sources of infection), and that rigorous measures are taken to ident[...] any infective organism—adequate blood cultures are key.

The diagnosis is usually based on a bacteraemia with a likely organism, coupled with evidence of cardiac involvement (e.g. new regurgitant lesion or vegetation). Investigations are therefore aimed at identifying these and also assessing severity and/or complications. There are situations however where other features may be helpful in reaching a diagnosis, and the widely accepted Duke criteria for diagnosis (see table) include these.

Investigations

Blood cultures

3–6 sets of blood cultures should be obtained: 3 when the patient is very unwell and the diagnosis of endocarditis is likely; 6 when the patient is well and the diagnosis not obvious but suspicion is high. Each set should be taken from a different site and, ideally, spaced at intervals >1 hr.

Echocardiography

Echocardiography should be performed if there is a high clinical suspicion of endocarditis (📖 p.99). It is invaluable for diagnosis and also detection of any complications. Strong identifiers of endocarditis are:
- Characteristic vegetations
- Abscesses
- New prosthetic valve dehiscence
- New regurgitation.

Transthoracic echocardiography (TTE) has high specificity for vegetations (98%) but low sensitivity (60%) and TOE may be required. Combined TTE and TOE have a high negative predictive value (95%) but note this is not 100%, and this underlines the importance of good clinical and microbiological evidence.

Native valves: TTE should be the initial investigation. TOE is required when the TTE images are of poor quality, when high clinical suspicion remains despite a normal TTE or when a prosthetic valve is involved.

Prosthetic valves: TOE is nearly always required for better visualisation but important information can still be obtained from TTE, so it is normal to perform this at the same time, just prior to the TOE.

Other investigations

Bloods: FBC—anaemia, neutrophilia, ESR, CRP—non-specific but raised in 90% of cases of endocarditis, U&E—renal function (needs regular repeat assessment), serum for immunology for atypical organisms.

Urinalysis: Microscopic haematuria ± proteinuria; Red cell casts & heavy proteinuria if glomerulonephritis.

ECG: Lengthening PR interval (?aortic root abscess).

...fied Duke criteria for diagnosis of endocarditis

...firmed diagnosis is based on either:

...thological criteria:	Organisms or histological evidence of active endocarditis in a vegetation (embolised or not) or intra-cardiac abscess.
Clinical criteria:	2 major criteria, or 1 major and 3 minor criteria, or 5 minor criteria.

Major criteria

Microbiological involvement—either:

- Typical microorganism for endocarditis from two separate blood cultures (Viridans streptococci; *Strep. bovis*; HACEK group¶, community acquired *S. aureus/enterococci* in the absence of a primary focus)
- Persistently positive blood cultures with consistent organisms (drawn >12 hrs apart, or ≥3 +ve cultures with first and last drawn >1 hr apart)
- Positive serology or molecular biology for Q-fever, *Coxiella burnettii* or other causes of culture-negative endocarditis.

Evidence of endocardial involvement:

- Oscillating intra-cardiac mass (vegetation)
- Abscess
- New partial dehiscence of prosthetic valve
- New valve regurgitation (either clinical or echocardiographic).

Minor criteria

- Predisposing heart condition or IV drug use
- Fever >38.0 °C
- Vascular phenomena (arterial emboli, septic pulmonary infarcts, mycotic aneurysm, intracranial or conjunctival haemorrhage, Janeway lesions, splinter haemorrhages, splenomegaly, newly diagnosed clubbing)
- Immunological phenomena (glomerulonephritis, Osler's nodes, Roth spots, +ve rheumatoid factor, high ESR >1.5 × normal, high CRP >100 mg/L)
- Microbiological evidence—+ve blood culture not meeting major criterion*, or serological evidence of active infection with organism consistent with infective endocarditis
- Echocardiography findings consistent with infective endocarditis but falling short of major criterion.

¶ Haemophilus, Acintobacillus, Cardiobacterium, Eikenella, and Kingella sp.
* Excludes single +ve culture for coagulase –ve Staph. and organisms not associated with infective endocarditis.

Treatment
General considerations
- ⚙: Treat heart failure and shock as appropriate
- Ensure blood cultures are taken prior to starting antibiotic therapy
- Give anti-microbial therapy in adequate doses IV for 4–6 weeks
- Monitor response to therapy—both clinically and biochemically
- Consider surgery if significant complications arise (📖 p.92).

Antimicrobial therapy
Uncomplicated cases: Treatment may be postponed for 48 hrs, allowing time for initial blood culture results. If the patient has had antibiotics within the last week, it is better to wait at least 48 hrs before taking blood cultures.

Severely unwell patients:—Sepsis, severe valve dysfunction, conduction disturbances, embolic events) should have empirical antibiotic therapy (see table) after 3 sets of blood cultures have been taken. Treatment can be adjusted once culture results are known.

Choice of therapy: This is guided by the organism but in all cases, microbiological advice should be sought early. Suggested regimes are in the table opposite, but these are for guidance only.

Treatment duration: In general this needs to be prolonged (4–6 weeks) IV therapy in adequate doses. Occasionally, shorter courses may be appropriate for the most sensitive streptococci only (see table). A tunnelled central line or peripherally inserted central catheter (PICC line) is usually inserted to facilitate IV therapy and reduce infections and other complications from repeated peripheral cannulae.

Prosthetic valve endocarditis
- Prosthetic (metal) valve endocarditis often requires replacement of the valve, though even then, recurrence rates are high (9–20%). This is due to the difficulty of eradicating infection from prosthetic material. Biological valves may be treated with antibiotics alone but need for surgery is still higher than for native valves
- Even with good TTE, TOE is required to visualise the valve properly due to the shadowing effect of the metal
- Prolonged antibiotic therapy is required (6 weeks)
- Warfarin is often replaced with heparin, for better control of anticoagulation and potential surgical situations.

Valve replacement surgery in endocarditis (📖 p.92)
- 30% require this during the acute episode—consider if valve function deteriorates enough to causes heart failure, infection remains uncontrolled despite adequate therapy or significant complications arise
- Although valve replacement surgery during active endocarditis does carry a risk of reinfection of the prosthesis, the risk is low and the risk to the patient (of death or irreversible LV dysfunction) if not operated on is higher for the indications given
- If cerebral emboli/haemorrhage have occurred, surgery should be deferred for 10 days–3 weeks if possible.

~~E~~mpirical treatment for endocarditis (if essential)

~~G~~uided by the clinical setting:

~~O~~nset over weeks:	Benzylpenicillin + gentamicin
Rapid onset (days) or history of skin trauma (likely staphylococcus):	Flucloxacillin + gentamicin
● Recent metal valve replacement:	Vancomycin + gentamicin + rifampicin.

Antibiotic therapy for known organism

—seek microbiological advice in all cases

Viridans streptococci and *Strep. Bovis*
● Benzylpenicillin 4–6 weeks + Gentamicin 2 weeks.

Staphylococci
● Methicillin-sensitive: Flucloxacillin 6 weeks + gentamicin 3–5 days
● Methicillin-resistant: Vancomycin 6 weeks + gentamicin 3–5 days
● Prosthetic valves: continue gentamicin for 6 weeks & add rifampicin 6 weeks.

Enterococci/HACEK group (the latter need amoxicillin)
● Benzylpenicillin/amoxicillin 4–6 weeks + Gentamicin 4–6 weeks.

Penicillin-allergic patients
● Vancomycin 4 weeks + gentamicin 2 weeks.

DOSES
● Benzylpenicillin—for streptococci, relies on minimum inhibitory concentration (MIC) of antibiotics required (i.e. sensitivity to penicillin):
  • MIC <0.1 mg/L: 7.2–12 g IV daily in 4–6 divided doses
  • MIC >0.1 mg/L (& enterococci): 12–14 g IV daily in 4–6 divided doses
● Gentamicin: 3–5mg/kg IV daily in 2–3 divided doses (max 240 mg/day)
  —requires blood level checking; dose is reduced in renal failure
● Flucloxacillin: 8–12 g IV daily in 4 divided doses
● Amoxicillin: 12 g IV daily in 4–6 divided doses
● Vancomycin: 30 mg/kg IV daily in 2 divided doses (infused over 2 hours)
● Rifampicin: 300 mg TDS po.

Shorter treatment regimes

May be possible if all the below apply:
● Infection with fully sensitive streptococcus (MIC <0.1 mg/L) on native valve
● Rapid response to treatment within 1st 7 days
● Any vegetations on echocardiography <10 mm
● No cardiovascular complications
● Home situation suitable.

Regimes possible
● Benzylpenicillin alone for 2 weeks (rarely, for exquisitely sensitive organisms)
● Benzylpenicillin alone for 1–2 weeks plus further 2 weeks ambulatory (home) treatment with ceftriaxone
● Benzylpenicillin + gentamicin for 2 weeks ± further 2 weeks ambulatory treatment with ceftriaxone.

Complications (esp. common with *S. aureus*)

Cardiac

- ① Abscesses (20–40% native valves; 50–100% prosthetic valves)—va. ring, intra-myocardial or pericardial. Usually require valve replacemen. surgery + debridement of the abscess
- ⚙ Valve rupture, perforation or regurgitation
- ⚙ Sinus of Valsalva rupture (2° to abscess). Requires emergency surgery
- ⚙ Ventricular septal defect (from myocardial abscess rupture)
- ⚙ LV failure—due to valve dysfunction or direct myocardial involvement
- ① AV heart block—due to aortic root abscess
- Relapse of endocarditis
- ⑦ Chronic valve regurgitation—if significant regurgitation occurs, but not enough to require urgent valve replacement, valve replacement may be required in the future (20–40% of cases). The indications are the same as for other causes of regurgitation (📖 p.92).

Non-cardiac

- ① **Emboli** (20–40%) → stroke, peripheral arterial occlusion, organ in-farcts. May also cause abscesses due to infected nature of embolic material. Abdominal abscesses should be operated on prior to cardiac surgery. Splenic abscesses are particularly prone to rupture and splenectomy may be required
- ① **Mycotic aneurysms** (2–15%)—often caused by embolised infected material. Common sites: sinuses of Valsalva, cerebral, mesenteric & renal arteries. Intra-cranial have high mortality (60%); increased if rupture occurs (→ sub-arachnoid haemorrhage: 80% mortality).
- ① **Renal failure** (sepsis, dehydration, glomerulonephritis, emboli).

Culture negative endocarditis (5% of cases)

Causes:

- Previous antibiotic therapy (the most common cause)
- Unusual organism—HACEK group, Brucella, Chlamydia, Coxiella (Q fever), Legionella, Bartonella, Mycobacteria, Nocardia, fungi (Candida, Aspergillus, Histoplasma).

Management

- Consider other (non-cardiac) causes for fever
- If high clinical suspicion for endocarditis remains:
  - Consult with microbiology regarding prolonged or special cultures; take serum for serology of unusual organisms
  - For unwell patients, treat empirically (📖 box p.103)
  - For well patients, await microbiological diagnosis
- If valve replacement surgery is required, the excised valve should be sent for culture and broad spectrum polymerase chain reaction (PCR) for DNA identification of organisms.

References

BCS guidelines (including detailed information on prophylaxis): available on the BCS website 17/1/05: www.bcs.com

ESC guidelines: Horstkotte D, Follath F, Gutschik E *et al.* (2004). *European Heart Journal* **25**, 267–276.

AHA guidelines: Bayer AS, Bolger AF, Taubert KA *et al.* (1998). *Circulation* **98**, 2936–2948.

Prosthetic valves

Types

Bioprosthetic

- Obtained from human cadavers (homograft), or manufactured from bovine or porcine pericardium (xenograft; e.g. Carpentier–Edwards). Pericardial valves may be suspended from 3 metal struts ('stented' valve) or contained within a covered wire frame (stentless)
- Do not require long term anticoagulation. Usually require 6 weeks of either warfarin or aspirin post-surgery while surfaces endothelialize
- Generally last 10–15 years—for this reason, are usually implanted in a) older patients, who also tend to be less active, reducing the physical burden on the valve, b) those in whom anticoagulation is contraindicated, and c) young women who may be considering pregnancy.

Metallic

- Three main sub-types:
  - Ball and cage (e.g. Starr–Edwards)—older style, unlikely to be implanted now. Durable, and long track record, but higher resistance to flow and high thrombogenicity
  - Single tilting disc (e.g. Bjork–Shiley, Medtronic Hall)
  - Bileaflet tilting disc (e.g. St. Jude, ATS 'Advancing The Standard')—commonest used today. Good track record, low resistance to flow, and low thrombogenicity
- Durable (can last >20 yrs) but thrombogenic, so require lifelong anticoagulation.

Clinical

- Bioprosthetic valves should sound little different from native valves, but pericardial valves may have a flow murmur
- ① Metallic valves have a distinctive 'click' as the valve either opens or closes. This should be a crisp sound—a dull or indistinct sound suggests thrombus or vegetation on the valve. Although flow murmurs may occur, these are soft. Other murmurs (pan-systolic, diastolic) suggest regurgitation
- All prosthetic valves require antibiotic prophylaxis prior to certain procedures (📖 p.96)
- Annual follow-up is routine for patients with prosthetic valves.

Echocardiography

Systolic flow velocities are in general increased with a normally-functioning prosthetic valve. Metal prostheses can have high velocities (>3 m/sec) and the normal range for that valve needs to be taken into account. The smaller the valve, the higher the forward velocity.

- **Biological:** Homografts look like normal valves; pericardial valves have a smaller valve ring in general and hence have slightly increased flow velocities, though the newer stentless type look virtually normal and have normal flow velocities
- **Metallic valves** cause echo 'shadows' which limit the available information. TOE may therefore be required on occasions to assess valve function in detail. For tilting-disc valves, it is normal to see tiny regurgitant 'wash' jets.

.etic valves

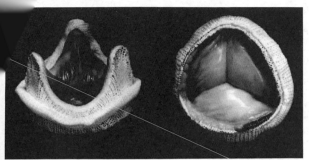

Carpentier–Edwards bioprosthetic valve

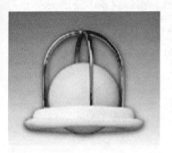

Ball and cage valve

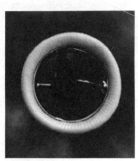

Single tilting disc valve

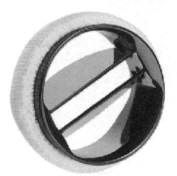

Bileaflet tilting valve

Complications
ⓘ *Thrombosis*
Usually from inadequate anticoagulation. Risk higher in mitral prost.
Present with heart failure or systemic emboli. Treat with heparin an̄
agulation ± thrombolysis, thrombectomy, or valve replacement.

ⓘ *Haemolysis*
Small amounts of haemolysis are common with metallic valves. Significant
haemolysis usually secondary to valve dysfunction—paravalvular leak,
valve dehiscence, or endocarditis. Bloods: anaemia, ↑reticulocyte count,
↑LDH, ↓haptoglobins. Urinary haemosiderin present. Treat the anaemia
with ferrous sulphate ± blood transfusions and the underlying cause—
may require re-do valve replacement surgery, though there are new
percutaneous devices for closing paravalvular leaks.

ⓘ *Endocarditis*
~5% patients with prosthetic valves may develop this.
- Early prosthetic valve endocarditis (<2 months post-implantation) is
  usually due to contamination at the time of surgery or IV cannulae.
  Common organisms: *S. aureus, S. epidermidis*, gram-negative bacteria,
  fungi
- Late prosthetic valve endocarditis has similar organisms to native valve
  endocarditis.

coagulation for metal valves—acute issues

general, the risk of thrombosis on a metal valve without anticoagula-
n for a few days is low, though should be minimised with heparin
where possible.

Emergency surgery

INR can be normalised with fresh frozen plasma to allow emergency
surgery. Once stable post-surgery, warfarin can be re-started.

Acute haemorrhage

In general, the risk to the patient of an acute haemorrhage (e.g. gastrointestinal or intracranial bleed) far outweighs the risk of thrombosis on
a metal valve and the warfarin should be reversed with fresh frozen
plasma ± vitamin K until the haemorrhagic risk has subsided. Even the
highest estimates of the risk of prosthetic valve thrombosis without any
anticoagulation are around 30–50% *per year* (~0.5–1% per week). The
short term bleeding risk in acute haemorrhage is usually much higher
than this, so the balance of risks is in favour of treating the haemorrhage and accepting a small risk of valve thrombosis.

Elective procedures requiring cessation of anticoagulation

- Some procedures (e.g. dental extraction) can be done with a
  lowering of the INR to ~2.5 rather than cessation of warfarin
- For surgery or other procedures where anticoagulation needs
  stopping, patients are normally admitted a few days in advance, and
  IV unfractionated heparin substituted for the warfarin. This can
  then be stopped a few hours prior to the surgery and re-started
  when the surgeon is happy the bleeding risk is low, minimising the
  time without anticoagulation. Low molecular weight heparin has not
  been adequately assessed for prosthetic valves and should be
  avoided. Warfarin can be restarted and the patient discharged once
  the INR is above 2.5.

ⓘ Acute rheumatic fever

- An immunologically-mediated systemic inflammatory illness, with significant cardiac component, several weeks following group A streptococcal infection (often a sore throat)
- Incidence now very rare in developed world, but common in Indian sub-continent, the Middle East, and Australian aboriginals
- Commonly affects children age 5–15, but long term damage to cardiac valves may result in problems in later life.

Presentation

Carditis

- Onset tends to be more insidious
- A pan-carditis can occur, with pericarditis, myocarditis & endocarditis:
  - Endocarditis, affecting the valves, is the most important aspect, and acute heart failure or chronic problems are usually due to this
  - Pericarditis ± effusion is common but rarely causes problems
  - Myocarditis may cause acute LV dysfunction, but this is rare
  - AV block (usually 1°)
- Regurgitant (esp. mitral) murmur is the commonest clinical feature.

Arthritis

- More rapid onset, over hours/days
- Large-joint, migratory polyarthritis (e.g. knees, ankles, wrists, elbows)
- Can be exquisitely painful—one joint tends to predominate.

Other

- Fever (common); abdominal pain (rare)
- Sydenham's chorea ('St. Vitus' dance')—rhythmic, involuntary upper limb movements. Usually after prolonged latent period (6 mo.) and resolves after 6 wks (occ. up to 6 mo.); usually affects females
- Subcutaneous nodules & erythema marginatum.

ΔΔ Infective arthritis; non-specific arthralgia in feverish child.

Treatment

- Bed rest until arthritis & any heart failure have resolved
- Penicillin for any remaining streptococci: penicillin G 1.2 MU single dose IM or penicillin V 250 mg po (adults 500 mg) tds for 10 days; erythromycin if penicillin-allergic—20–40 mg/kg/d (adults 250 mg qds)
- Aspirin or other NSAIDS for arthritis (usually high dose: 80–100 mg/kg/d; adults 4–8 g/d, in divided doses)
- ? Corticosteroids—often still used, but evidence for benefit is low; prednisolone 40–60 mg/d, tapering after 2–3 wks
- Treat heart failure; consider valve replacement if severe dysfunction
- Haloperidol or other drugs for chorea.

Prevention of recurrence

2° prophylaxis is required—penicillin V 250 mg bd (or IM penicillin G 1.2 MU every 3 wks). Minimum duration: 5 yrs or until age 21 (whichever is later); if severe valve destruction, continue to age 30 or more.

...ed Jones criteria for diagnosis of initial attack of ...e rheumatic fever (1992)*

...nosis requires both:

...emonstration of current/recent group A streptococcal infection.

(culture or serological tests e.g. anti-streptolysin O. Chorea and late-onset carditis are exempt.)

> And

2 major, or 1 major plus 2 minor criteria:

Major Criteria
- Carditis
- Polyarthritis
- Chorea
- Subcutaneous nodules
- Erythema marginatum.

Minor Criteria
- Fever
- Arthralgia
- Elevated acute phase reactants
- Prolonged PR interval.

* Recurrent attacks require only 1 major or 2 minor criteria, plus evidence of recent Gp A streptococcus and no other explanation for symptoms.

Valve disease in acute rheumatic fever

Affected valves
Mitral (65–70%), aortic (25%), tricuspid (10%, with other valves), pulmonary (rare).

Acute effects
Inflammation, destruction, and valve regurgitation.

Long term effects
(30–50%; 70% if severe carditis during acute phase):
- Regurgitation
- Stenosis due to scarring and contraction following the acute inflammation
- Valves typically appear thickened, with rolled edges and tips on echocardiography.

Valve repair
If valve surgery required, valves might be suitable for repair during the acute episode, but are usually unsuitable for repair in the chronic stage.

Aortic stenosis

The commonest valve lesion; prevalence 2% >65yrs of age.

Causes
- Degenerative (most common)
- Bicuspid aortic valve (may be accelerated degeneration). Bicuspid valves also have an association with both coarctation and aortic dilatation ± dissection, even in the absence of aortic valve dysfunction
- Previous rheumatic fever.

Clinical features
Symptoms
- May be none
- SOB, syncope or angina may all occur and signify poor prognosis.

Signs
- Harsh, musical, ejection systolic murmur best heard in aortic region, radiating to carotids
- If severe: slow-rising pulse, heaving non-displaced apex, soft or absent 2nd heart sound
- LV hypertrophy on ECG.

ΔΔ Sub-aortic obstruction, hypertrophic obstructive cardiomyopathy.

Acute problems
① Acute presentation of chronic disease
- Symptom onset can be rapid (days/weeks) and should prompt consideration for aortic valve replacement (AVR)
- If LV function poor, may be in intractable pulmonary oedema—AVR is the only treatment. Many patients improve if they survive surgery.

① Acute stenosis
- Rare
- Causes: thrombus on prosthetic valve, vegetation
- Usually requires prompt AVR.

Treatment
Aortic valve replacement
This is the only real 'cure' and is performed if symptomatic severe AS.

Medical (for temporary relief)
- SOB can be treated with diuretics
- Beta-blockers may be useful, particularly for angina
- Vasodilator drugs should be used cautiously.

Balloon valvuloplasty
May be used in younger patients (less calcified valve) as a holding measure to defer surgery (e.g. if pregnant).

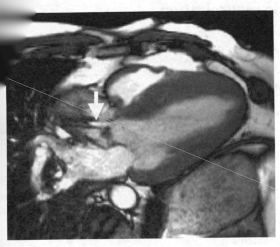

Cardiac magnetic resonance image of severe aortic stenosis, demonstrating a high velocity eccentric jet of aortic flow.

Aortic regurgitation

Causes
Acute: Type A aortic dissection, aortic valve endocarditis, trauma.
Chronic: Previous infective endocarditis, aortic root dilatation (includir
Marfan syndrome), degenerative valve, previous rheumatic fever.

Clinical features
- Acute AR causes sudden severe SOB and pulmonary oedema
- In severe chronic disease, SOB may be the only symptom.

Signs
- Early diastolic, decrescendo murmur heard at the lower left sternal edge, best in expiration
- ± Ejection systolic flow murmur (increased forward flow across valve)
- In severe disease:
  - Collapsing pulse
  - Displaced, hyperdynamic apex (due to dilated LV)
  - Other eponymous signs, mostly due to widened pulse pressure (see box).

Acute problems
:☼: *Acute (sudden) regurgitation*
- Patient is extremely unwell, and often in pulmonary oedema
- Needs emergency valve replacement (± aortic root replacement if dissection)
- Holding treatments while surgery arranged: diuretics, vasodilators, inotropes, ventilation. (NOT intra-aortic balloon pump as this worsens the AR).

Acute presentation of chronic disease
Once symptoms develop in chronic disease, aortic valve replacement should be considered, so these patients fall into this category.

Mixed aortic valve disease

- *Causes:* Bicuspid valve, rheumatic heart disease, endocarditis on aortic stenosis, previous (partially successful) valvuloplasty for stenosis
- True mixed aortic valve disease should be differentiated from aortic regurgitation with ↑systolic aortic flow velocity 2° to ↑stroke volume, and from aortic stenosis with a mild leak (not uncommon)
- The relative severity of each component (stenosis/regurgitation) is variable, though predominant stenosis is more common and is the more significant problem
- The combination of a narrowed outlet and need for increased stroke volume places substantial demands on the myocardium, and the LV is often very hypertrophied and responds poorly to rapid changes. Acute problems can therefore occur more readily, e.g. deterioration with the onset of AF.

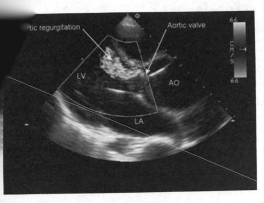

Parasternal transthoracic echocardiogram demonstrating a broad jet of aortic regurgitation in a patient with a dilated aorta (AO).

Eponymous signs in severe AR

Sign	Clinical features
Corrigan's	Visible carotid pulsation.
de Musset's	Head bobbing with each pulse.
Müller's	Visible uvula pulsation.
Quincke's	Visible capillary pulsation in nailbed.
Traube's	Systolic & diastolic femoral sounds ('pistol-shot' femorals).
Duroziez's	Compression of femoral artery proximally causes systolic bruit; distal compression causes proximal bruit.

Mitral stenosis

Incidence has significantly declined in developed countries due to reduction in its major cause, rheumatic fever.

Causes
- Previous rheumatic fever
- Other rare causes: congenital, bulky vegetation, atrial myxoma.

Clinical features

Acute mitral stenosis is extraordinarily rare. Most present chronically—insidious onset, with SOB, fatigue or reduced exercise tolerance.
Signs: AF not uncommon, malar flush, prominent a waves in JVP.
Auscultation: Prominent S1, opening snap, low-pitched mid-diastolic rumbling murmur with pre-systolic accentuation (atrial contraction).
ECG: Bifid P wave (± peaked P wave if pulmonary HT), AF.

ⓘ Acute problems
- Often caused by ↑heart rate. This is tolerated badly due to the increased time required for passage of blood across the stenotic valve
- Common causes: AF, exercise, infection (esp. chest), pregnancy
- Present with SOB ± heart failure.

ⓘ Atrial fibrillation
With acute AF, the loss of atrial contraction in addition to the sudden increase in heart rate can rapidly precipitate heart failure.

Treatment
ⓘ The combination of heart failure and mod–severe mitral stenosis is difficult to treat and expert help should be sought urgently.
- Diuretics
- Rate control (digoxin for AF; diltiazem/verapamil, beta-blockers)—this is a difficult balance in a patient with heart failure
- Consider cardioversion for acute AF (not useful for chronic)
- ?Balloon valvuloplasty.

Longer term issues

Atrial fibrillation
Permanent AF is common in mitral stenosis and rate control is required.

▶ Anticoagulation is vital—thrombotic risk is huge (11× other AF).

Surgery—for symptoms, or pulmonary hypertension. Options:
- Closed valvotomy (separation of fused cusps)
- Open valvotomy (on cardiac bypass)
- Mitral valve replacement.

Balloon valvuloplasty
- For valves without significant calcification or regurgitation
- Can give moderate relief for several months/years but restenosis usually occurs
- Particularly good for acute presentations in pregnancy.

Mitral regurgitation

Causes

The mitral valve is a complex structure, relying on the papillary m
chordae and myocardial motion for its effective function. Intrinsic
disease may not therefore be the only cause of dysfunction, and o.
reasons should be excluded.

Acute: Infective endocarditis, MI (papillary muscle infarction, rupture, o
tethering to infarcted LV wall), ruptured chordae tendinae, trauma.

Chronic: Degenerative disease, mitral prolapse, dilated LV, myocardial
dysfunction 2° to ischaemia, previous rheumatic fever.

Clinical features

Symptoms
- Acute MR causes sudden, severe SOB and pulmonary oedema
- Chronic disease may be asymptomatic for many years
- In severe chronic disease, SOB may be the only symptom and should
  prompt consideration of valve replacement.

Signs
- Pan-systolic murmur (soft, blowing) at apex, radiating to axilla
- If severe:
  - Wide splitting of S2, due to early aortic valve closure
  - Loud S3
  - Displaced, hyperdynamic apex.

Acute problems

:۞: *Acute (sudden) regurgitation*
- Commonest cause is post-MI (papillary muscle involvement)
- Patient is extremely unwell, and often in pulmonary oedema
- Needs emergency valve replacement/repair (?of papillary muscle)
- Holding treatments while surgery arranged: diuretics, inotropes,
  vasodilators, ventilation, intra-aortic balloon pump.

① *Acute presentation of chronic disease*

Like aortic regurgitation, once symptoms develop in chronic disease,
valve replacement/repair should be considered, but it is important to
exclude a 'functional' cause for MR such as a dilated LV with poor function, or ischaemia, as these should be treated directly.

In chronic MR, left ventricular pressure is 'off-loaded' by the flow of
blood into the low pressure left atrium. Therefore the function should
appear good and, in severe MR, vigorous. A 'normal' or slightly reduced
ejection fraction in the presence of severe MR may thus in fact represent
early LV dysfunction. Systolic LV dilation on echocardiography (>4.5 cm)
is a good indicator of LV dysfunction.

> **Mitral prolapse (floppy mitral valve)**
> - Mostly idiopathic, prevalence 5–10% of the population
> - If no or trivial regurgitation is present, does not need follow up
> - ≥ mild regurgitation needs follow-up and endocarditis prophylaxis
> - Symptoms from ectopic beats. Reports of atypical chest pain are inconsistent
> - Classical late-systolic murmur if regurgitation present
> - Can degenerate to severe mitral regurgitation requiring surgery.

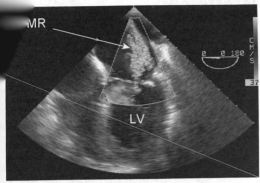

Transoesophageal echocardiogram demonstrating mitral regurgitation.

Surgery in mitral regurgitation

Valve replacement
For intrinsic, severe disease unsuitable for repair. Metal prostheses are used—bioprosthetic valves tend to degenerate quickly, and are not routinely placed in the mitral position.

Valve repair
For severe MR 2° to prolapse, where the valve anatomy is otherwise reasonably normal. Rheumatic and other damaged valves are not usually suitable. Posterior leaflet repair is much more successful than anterior, though it is a technically demanding operation and both types require an experienced surgeon. Even in the best hands, repair is not always successful, and replacement is the fall-back position. Long term results are good in selected cases, and minimally-invasive repair, utilising robotic arms, has been successful in a handful of cases to date.

Valve ring insertion
For cases where the mitral annulus is enlarged, causing failure of coaption of the leaflets (either LV or LA enlargement). A 'C' shaped ring is sewn around the valve to reduce the annular size and restore integrity of function. Commonly combined with valve repair for prolapse with dilated LA/LV and with CABG for ischaemic, dilated LV and functional regurgitation.

Papillary muscle repair
In cases of papillary rupture (usually secondary to MI), re-attachment of the papillary muscle may be all that is required for restoration of valve function. CABG may be performed at the same sitting, to deal with the coronary stenosis, but this depends on the clinical situation.

Pulmonary stenosis

Causes

Congenital (may be in conjunction with other defects e.g. Fallot's te...ogy), rheumatic fever, carcinoid.

Clinical features

Few symptoms—SOB if severe.
Signs: RV heave, prominent a wave in JVP ± tricuspid regurgitation, quiet P2, soft ejection systolic murmur at upper left sternal edge.
ECG: RVH, P pulmonale.

Acute problems

Rare—rapid increase in heart rate can lead to right-sided heart failure.

Treatment

- Balloon valvuloplasty. Usual first-line treatment. Effective and may be repeated in future. Pulmonary regurgitation is the main side effect and is usually tolerated well
- Surgical (open) valvotomy—very effective with good long term results
- Pulmonary valve replacement (rarely required).

Pulmonary regurgitation

Causes

Congenital, endocarditis, 2° to pulmonary hypertension, following balloon valvuloplasty or open valvotomy.

Clinical features

Tolerated extremely well mostly. SOB if v. severe, or RV failure occurs.
Signs: RV heave, loud ± delayed P2, ± soft pulmonary ejection murmur, diastolic decrescendo murmur at mid left sternal edge, RV failure.
ECG: RVH.

Acute problems

Rare—RV failure may develop and present acutely; acute pulmonary hypertension (e.g. from pulmonary embolus) may cause PR.

Treatment

- Usually none required (tolerated v. well)
- Treat any RV failure
- Treat cause of pulmonary hypertension
- If severe symptoms and RV failure, pulmonary valve replacement can be considered
- New techniques include a bioprosthetic valve mounted on a stent, which can be inserted percutaneously in the pulmonary position.

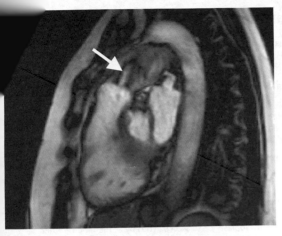

Cardiac magnetic resonance image showing the RV outflow tract. There is significant pulmonary stenosis (arrow indicates high velocity jet).

Tricuspid stenosis

Causes
Rheumatic fever (usually in association with mitral stenosis), carcir.
very rarely with a pacemaker lead.

Clinical features
Fatigue.

Signs: Raised JVP with prominent 'a' wave, mid-diastolic murmur at left
sternal edge—similar to mitral stenosis but higher pitch, hepatomegaly
and peripheral oedema if severe.

Acute problems
• Almost never
• Acute stenosis could occur with large infective vegetation.

Treatment
• Diuretics
• Balloon valvuloplasty or surgical valvotomy at the time of other
  (usually mitral) lesions are dealt with
• Valve replacement is avoided due to the difficulty with low right-sided
  venous pressures and the resistance to flow from a prosthetic valve.

Tricuspid regurgitation

Causes
Congenital (incl. Ebstein's anomaly), Marfan's, any cause of RV dilatation,
pulmonary hypertension, endocarditis, carcinoid.

Clinical features
• Minimal symptoms
• Right heart failure can develop if severe
• *Signs:* Large 'v' waves in JVP, pulsatile hepatomegaly, (peripheral
  oedema, ascites ± jaundice if significant RV failure), very soft
  pan-systolic murmur at left sternal edge.

Acute problems
• Rare
• Tricuspid endocarditis may occur in IV drug users, and is usually
  staphylococcal. It follows an aggressive course and needs intensive
  antibiotic treatment.

Treatment
• Usually none required
• Diuretics are the mainstay of treatment for symptoms and RV failure
• Tricuspid valvuloplasty, annuloplasty, and valve replacement are rarely
  undertaken and long term results are disappointing.

Arrhythmias

Brachyarrhythmias
Bradycardia *126*
Sinus bradycardia *126*
Sinus arrest *128*
Junctional bradycardia *130*
Atrioventricular block *132*
Tachyarrhythmias
Tachycardia *136*
Sinus tachycardia *138*
Atrial fibrillation *140*
Atrial flutter *144*
Atrial tachycardia *148*
Atrioventricular nodal reentrant tachycardia (AVNRT) *150*
Atrioventricular reentrant tachycardia (AVRT) *152*
Ventricular fibrillation (VF) *154*
Ventricular tachycardia (VT) *156*
Monomorphic ventricular tachycardia *156*
Polymorphic ventricular tachycardia
    ('Torsade de Pointes') *160*
Electrical storms *162*
The ICD in the emergency room *164*
Commonly used antiarrhythmic agents
    in the emergency setting *166*

Bradycardia

- A heart rate of less than 60 beat/minute.

Bradycardia may occur as a normal physiological variant, secondary disease process or as a result of drug therapy. Presentations include coincidental finding in the asymptomatic patient, fatigue, breathlessness on exertion, pre-syncope, or syncope. Bradycardia may be intermittent or persistent. The site of conduction disturbance may be the sinoatrial node, atrioventricular (AV) node or His–Purkinje system. Immediate management depends upon the degree of haemodynamic compromise, coexisting medical conditions, the site of conduction disturbance and prognostic implications.

ⓘ Sinus bradycardia

Symptoms
- Asymptomatic, coincidental finding, especially if nocturnal
- Fatigue
- Exertional dyspnoea
- Less commonly, pre-syncope or syncope.

Causes
- Physiological (fit, young patients at rest) in which case it is asymptomatic
- Drug treatment (e.g. beta-blockers)
- Systemic illness (e.g. hypothyroidism, hypothermia)
- Sinus node disease.

Immediate management
- Assess haemodynamic status (blood pressure, level of consciousness, urine output, signs of heart failure)
- Identify causative factors (drug history, thyroid status, electrolytes)
- If haemodynamically compromised: give atropine 1 mg IV.

Prognosis and subsequent management
- Good prognosis
- Irreversible, symptomatic bradycardia may require permanent pacemaker insertion.

Specific considerations
- It is very rare to require temporary transvenous pacing for sinus bradycardia, although it may be required for severe haemodynamic compromise in bradycardia that can not be treated pharmacologically
- Beta-blocker or calcium channel blocker overdose (📖 p.264).

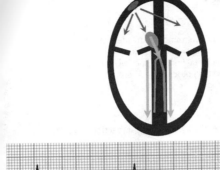

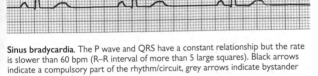

Sinus bradycardia. The P wave and QRS have a constant relationship but the rate is slower than 60 bpm (R–R interval of more than 5 large squares). Black arrows indicate a compulsory part of the rhythm/circuit, grey arrows indicate bystander (non-participating) pathways.

① Sinus arrest

Presentation
- Sinus arrest is often intermittent with an adequate rhythm and haemodynamic status in between episodes
- Asymptomatic, coincidental finding, especially if nocturnal (*sinus arrest is only 'significant' if pauses are >3 seconds*)
- Pre-syncope or syncope.

Causes
- Intrinsic sinus node disease
- Carotid sinus hypersensitivity or vasovagal reaction (📖 p.32).

Immediate management
- Dictated by frequency and severity of pauses
- Stop potentially exacerbating medications (beta-blockers, calcium channel blockers)
- Usually no immediate management is required even though a permanent pacemaker may be indicated
- Very frequent pauses resulting in severe symptoms may require temporary transvenous pacing.

Prognosis and subsequent management
- Good prognosis
- Symptomatic sinus arrest may require permanent pacemaker insertion.

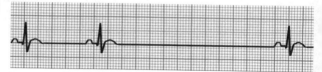

Sinus arrest. The P waves slows or stop suddenly, resulting in a pause. Significant pauses are those >3 seconds, particularly when the patient is awake.

⑦ Junctional bradycardia

Junctional bradycardia occurs when the sinus node fails and a low a. or AV junction pacemaker takes over. Retrograde P waves (negative lead II) may be visible immediately before, within or after the QRS com plex, which may be narrow or broad (ECG 📖 p.327). Symptoms resul. from a bradycardia and loss of the atrial contribution to ventricular filling, particularly if atrial and ventricular contractions are simultaneous.

Presentation
- Asymptomatic, coincidental finding, especially if nocturnal
- Fatigue
- Exertional dyspnoea
- Less commonly, pre-syncope or syncope.

Causes
- Drug treatment (e.g. beta-blockers, calcium channel blockers)
- Systemic illness (e.g. hypothyroidism, hypothermia)
- Hypokalaemia
- Sinus node disease with junctional escape.

Immediate management
- Assess haemodynamic status (blood pressure, level of consciousness, urine output, signs of heart failure)
- Identify causative factors (drug history, thyroid status, electrolytes)
- If haemodynamically compromised: give atropine 1 mg IV.

Prognosis and subsequent management
- Good prognosis
- Irreversible, symptomatic bradycardia may require permanent pacemaker insertion.

Specific considerations
Temporary transvenous pacing for junctional bradycardia may be required for severe haemodynamic compromise. Single chamber ventricular pacing may not improve cardiac output and atrial or dual chamber AV sequential pacing may be required (📖 p.296).

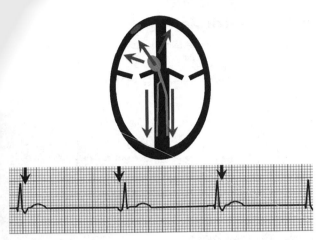

Junctional bradycardia. If the sinus node pacemaker fails, the AV junction is next in line in the pacemaker hierarchy. P waves originate from the AV node area and are therefore negative in leads II, III and aVF. They occur just before, during or after the QRS (arrows), depending upon which point in the AV junction they originate. There is a QRS complex, usually narrow, for every P wave. Black arrows indicate a compulsory part of the rhythm/circuit, grey arrows indicate bystander (non-participating) pathways.

⑦ Atrioventricular block

Conduction delay or block between the atria and the ventricles m.
within the AV node (usually narrow QRS complex, benign, and respe
to increase in sympathetic tone) or the His–Purkinje system (QRS m.
be wide, worse prognosis and doesn't respond to autonomic changes).

Classification

1° AV block

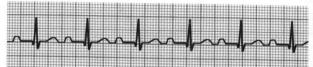

The PR interval is greater than 200 ms (1 large square). There is a QRS after every
P wave.

2° AV block (ECG 📖 p.328)

• Mobitz Type I (Wenckebach)

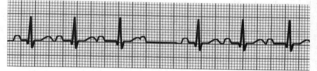

The PR interval lengthens after each successive P wave until finally one P wave is
not conducted.

• Mobitz Type II

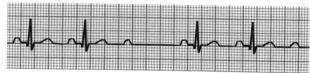

P waves fail to conduct to the ventricle in a fixed ratio without preceding
lengthening or variation in the PR interval.

3°/complete AV block (ECG 📖 p.329)

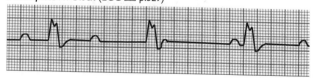

All P waves fail to conduct to the ventricle, resulting in a slow, dissociated ventricular escape rhythm. QRS complexes may be narrow or wide depending upon the
site of the escape rhythm origin.

...ntation

- ..mptomatic, coincidental finding
- ..tigue, exertional dyspnoea, or low cardiac output state
- ..resyncope or syncope.

..auses

- High vagal tone (usually benign and asymptomatic, usually has a narrow complex escape rhythm)
- Primary conduction tissue disease
- Myocardial disease (ischaemia, infarction, fibrosis, infiltration)—usually affects His–Purkinje system and had a wide complex escape rhythm
- Congenital
- Drugs (e.g. beta-blocker and calcium channel blocker combination).

Immediate management

1° degree and Mobitz type I 2° degree (Wenckebach) block do not normally require urgent intervention. Mobitz type II and complete AV block may require assessment for temporary transvenous pacing.

- Treat any precipitating causes (acute MI, drug overdose, abnormal electrolytes)
- Atropine (1 mg IV) will improve AV node conduction in the setting of high vagal tone but will have little effect on conduction disturbances due to His–Purkinje disease. Effects may last up to 3 hours
- Intravenous isoprenaline or other sympathomimetic drugs rarely improve conduction
- ① Temporary pacing is required for Mobitz type II 2° degree block or complete heart block if there is a low cardiac output state with reduced perfusion or recurrent syncope
- Complete heart block with mild or infrequent symptoms may be observed until permanent pacing is performed, especially if the QRS complex is narrow.

Prognosis and subsequent management

- Discontinue exacerbating antiarrhythmic medications
- Good prognosis if due to AV nodal block (narrow QRS, escape rhythm >45 bpm) and reversible cause
- Irreversible Mobitz type II 2° degree block or complete heart block due to His–Purkinje disease has an increased mortality and usually requires permanent pacemaker insertion, whether symptomatic or not.

① Myocardial infarction and AV block

Inferior MI

In the setting of acute inferior MI, thrombolysis or primary angiopla.
should not be delayed by complete heart block unless the patient
severely haemodynamically compromised. Heart block is usually tran
sient and reperfusion often results in restoration of normal conduction.
If conduction returns to normal within 48 hours, permanent pacemaker
insertion is not usually required. Temporary pacing is rarely required
and occasionally recovery of AV conduction can take over a week.

Anterior MI

Complete heart block in the setting of acute anterior MI carries a poor
prognosis and insertion of a temporary transvenous pacing wire should
be considered.

Atrioventricular block and AF or flutter

High grade AV block may result in symptoms due to a slow ventricular
response, either persistent bradycardia or symptomatic pauses. Pauses
(R–R intervals) of less than 3 seconds are not significant (particularly at
night).

Causes

- Intrinsic conduction tissue disease
- Coexisting cardiac disease (ischaemia, infarction, fibrosis, infiltration)
- Drugs (particularly beta-blocker and calcium channel blocker
  combination).

Immediate management

- Treat any precipitating causes (acute MI, drug overdose, abnormal
  electrolytes)
- Atropine (1 mg IV) will improve AV node conduction in the setting of
  high vagal tone but will have little effect on conduction disturbances
  due to His–Purkinje disease
- ① Temporary pacing is required only if there is a low cardiac output
  state with reduced perfusion or recurrent syncope. Slow ventricular
  rates with mild or infrequent symptoms may be observed until permanent pacing is performed.

Prognosis and subsequent management

- Discontinue exacerbating antiarrhythmic medications
- Irreversible high grade AV block due to His–Purkinje disease has
  an increased mortality and usually requires permanent pacemaker
  insertion, whether symptomatic or not.

Tachycardia

A heart rate of more than 100 beats/minute. Usually subdivided into:
- Narrow complex (regular, QRS duration <120 ms)
- Broad complex (regular, QRS complex >120 ms)
- AF with rapid ventricular response (irregular rhythm, may be narrow or broad complex).

Diagnosis should always be made using a 12-lead ECG, not telemetry as a true wide complex tachycardia may appear narrow in some leads.

▶▶ ☼: Look for haemodynamic compromise—reduced conscious level, hypotension, pulmonary oedema, cardiac ischaemia, poor perfusion. Requires immediate restoration of sinus rhythm with cardioversion under sedation or general anaesthesia.

▶ ☼: Look for underlying cause that may need urgent treatment—acute myocardial infarction, acute pulmonary embolism, severe electrolyte abnormality.

ECG diagnosis of broad complex tachycardia
▶ **A broad complex tachycardia should be assumed to be VT until proven otherwise.**

The following ECG criteria confirm a diagnosis of VT:
- *AV dissociation:* Manifest as independent P wave activity, fusion beats or capture beats (ECG 🕮 p.337). Be aware that slow VT, or idiopathic VT in a young person, may have 1:1 conduction retrogradely into the atrium
- *QRS duration >160 ms:* VT originating from the intraventricular septum may be relatively narrow with QRS 130–150 ms
- *Superior axis* (–45 to –135 degrees) and RBBB-type QRS shape
- *Inferior axis* (60 to 120 degrees) and LBBB-type QRS shape
- Onset of R wave to deepest point of S wave >100 ms in any chest lead
- *Concordance* across the chest leads (all QRS complexes predominantly positive or predominantly negative).

An ECG in sinus rhythm is helpful if it demonstrates bundle branch block that is identical to the wide complex tachycardia QRS shape. However, ECG evidence of prior MI makes the diagnosis of VT very likely.

Clinically, the rate and the degree of haemodynamic compromise are not good discriminators.

The presence of structural heart disease and/or a history of ischaemic heart disease are strong predictors of a diagnosis of VT.

▶ If in doubt, it is safer to mistreat an SVT as VT rather than treat a VT as an SVT.

The role of intravenous adenosine
- Adenosine is a very short-acting intravenous drug that specifically blocks the specialized conducting tissue of the AV node, with lesser effects on the sinus node and atrial myocardium
- The principle effect is to cause transient AV nodal block. Any tachycardia dependent on AV node conduction will therefore terminate when AV node block occurs
- Tachycardias that are not dependent on AV node conduction for their maintenance (AF, flutter) will continue, although the ECG appearance may transiently change, aiding diagnosis

...ctopic atrial tachycardias and idiopathic VTs may however also
...minated with adenosine
...wise, on rare occasions AV nodal dependent arrhythmias may
...minate, but reinitiate after a few beats of sinus rhythm
...gh doses of adenosine may induce AF in 5–10% of patients
• Adenosine administration often results in ventricular ectopy but it is
  rare for it to provoke sustained VT.

Administration
▶ Always record a continuous ECG immediately before, during and after
adenosine administration.
• Administer as a rapid intravenous bolus through a large cannula placed
  as centrally as possible
• Follow immediately by at least 10 mL flush of saline
• It is best to connect the adenosine and flush syringes to the cannula
  through a three-way tap to facilitate administration
• Start with a 6 mg bolus, and if there is no effect, increase to 12 mg,
  and in large patients, consider 18 mg or higher
• Patients will experience transient chest tightness, sweating and
  flushing during administration. Warn them.

Contraindications
• Severe asthma (adenosine is reported to be safe in mild asthmatics)
• Dipyridamole use (inhibits adenosine uptake and potentiates its effect)
• Caution with severe sinus node disease, cardiac transplant recipients
• To reverse the effects of adenosine, give aminophylline IV.

Arrhythmia	Effect of adenosine
Sinus tachycardia	Transient slowing of sinus rate. Transient AV block with ongoing P waves. As adenosine wears off sinus tachycardia rate may increase.
Atrial tachycardia	60% will show transient AV block with ongoing P waves. In some cases the atrial rate may also transiently slow. 10% of automatic atrial tachycardias are adenosine sensitive and will terminate. No effect in the remainder.
Atrial fibrillation	Transient AV block. Fibrillatory baseline still visible up until AV conduction returns.
Atrial flutter	Transient AV block. Flutter waves become clearly visible up until AV conduction returns.
AV nodal re-entrant tachycardia	Tachycardia terminates and sinus rhythm returns.
AV re-entrant tachycardia	Tachycardia terminates and sinus rhythm returns.
Atrial fibrillation and pre-excitation through accessory pathway	❶ QRS complexes transiently widen and ventricular rate may increase further, possibly resulting in ventricular fibrillation.
Ventricular tachycardia	Usually no effect, however some idiopathic ventricular tachycardias in normal hearts may terminate.

⑦ Sinus tachycardia

- Sinus tachycardia is a physiological response, usually to physical or emotional stress
- The rate is typically 100–160 bpm and is not constant but has subtle variation
- There is almost always an identifiable underlying cause
- Inappropriate sinus tachycardia is a rare condition marked by a dramatic increases in heart rate with minimal exertion and a mean resting rate >100 bpm
- Sinus node reentrant tachycardia is also rare and may mimic sinus tachycardia but often has a sudden onset and termination and responds to IV adenosine.

Principle causes
- Pain
- Anxiety
- Sepsis
- Hypoxia (asthma, PE, pulmonary oedema)
- Shock
- Anaemia
- Inotrope infusions
- Thyrotoxicosis.

ECG diagnosis
At rapid rates the P wave may be hard to identify, but there are often discrete P waves that are the same shape as those present in sinus rhythm (positive in lead II). There is usually a normal PR interval and 1:1 conduction to the ventricles.

Treatment
Identify and treat the underlying cause.

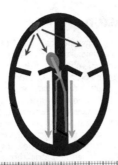

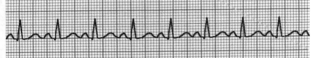

Sinus tachycardia. The P wave is a normal shape and axis and precedes each QRS with a normal PR interval. There are often subtle variations in the heart rate. Black arrows indicate a compulsory part of the rhythm/circuit, grey arrows indicate bystander (non-participating) pathways.

Atrial fibrillation (AF)

- The commonest clinical arrhythmia, affecting 1% of the population
- Symptoms result from a rapid, irregular ventricular rate and loss of atrial contribution to ventricular filling and cardiac output
- Patients may be asymptomatic, have palpitation, chest pain, dyspnoea, presyncope, syncope, or frank pulmonary oedema
- AF may be *paroxysmal* (will spontaneously revert to sinus rhythm), *persistent* (requires pharmacologic or electrical cardioversion to restore sinus rhythm) or *permanent* (sinus rhythm can not be restored)
- The thromboembolic risk that results from the development of AF and the restoration of sinus rhythm needs to be considered when assessing the various treatment strategies. Left atrial thrombus results from loss of atrial contractility and increased stasis and pooling of blood in the left atrial appendage. Restoration of sinus rhythm restores atrial contractile function and may result in embolism of any atrial thrombus present. This risk should be considered the same whether electrical or pharmacological cardioversion has occurred.

Principle causes

Idiopathic, hypertension, mitral valve disease, cardiomyopathy (ischaemic, dilated or hypertrophic), acute infection, thyrotoxicosis, post-surgery.

ECG diagnosis

Irregular ventricular rhythm. No discrete atrial activity (although lead V1 often has a coarse, rapid fibrillatory baseline). ECG 📖 p.330.

Treatment—general principles

- The two principal strategies are restoration of sinus rhythm or ventricular rate control. Some pharmacological treatments may address both
- If the duration of AF is greater than 48 hours there is an increased thromboembolic risk associated with restoration of sinus rhythm
- If AF has been present for more than 48 hours, cardioversion should therefore only be performed if the patient is on long-term effective anticoagulation, or has had a transoesophageal echocardiogram to exclude left atrial thrombus, or is haemodynamically compromised and the benefits of cardioversion outweigh the thromboembolic risks
- If patients present with shorter than 48 hours of AF, the dilemma is between waiting to see if AF stops spontaneously, or attempt immediate cardioversion before the 48 hour time limit is reached. As long as systemic anticoagulation is started with heparin, there is time to assess the patient and make a decision based upon symptoms, haemodynamic status and general practicalities.

▶ If the duration of AF is unknown, assume it is greater than 48 hours.

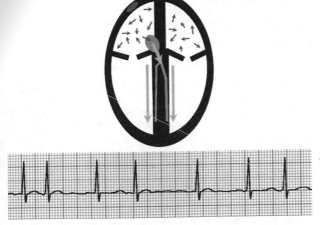

AF. Irregular QRS complexes. No obvious discrete P wave activity, although it is not unusual to see more organized activity in lead V1 with sharp bumps every 4–6 small squares. Black arrows indicate a compulsory part of the rhythm/circuit, grey arrows indicate bystander (non-participating) pathways.

☼ 1. AF with severe haemodynamic compromise

Ventricular rate >150 bpm, hypotension and hypoperfusion, r conscious level, pulmonary oedema, cardiac ischaemia.

- Oxygen
- Heparin IV (5–10,000 iu)
- Synchronized DC shock under sedation/general anaesthesia using 200–360 J monophasic or 150–200 J biphasic energy.

① 2. Symptomatic AF with mild-moderate haemodynamic compromise

Ventricular rate 100–150 bpm, breathless and/or mild hypotension. Consider other causes for haemodynamic compromise e.g. sepsis.

Onset <48 hours

- Heparin (5–10,000 iu IV) then subcutaneous low-molecular weight
- Consider pharmacological cardioversion with amiodarone 300 mg IV over 1 hour
- If the patient has good haemodynamics, no pulmonary oedema and no known structural heart disease (no previous ischaemic heart disease or valve disease and a normal transthoracic echocardiogram) an alternative to amiodarone is flecainide 2 mg/kg (max 150 mg) IV over 30 minutes. Plan for electrical cardioversion 2 to 3 hours later if drug treatment fails
- Synchronized DC shock under sedation/general anaesthesia using 200–360 J monophasic or 150 J biphasic energy
- If immediate electrical cardioversion is not available, start treatment with amiodarone while waiting.

Onset >48 hours

- Low molecular weight heparin subcutaneously
- Rate control with one of the following:
  - Digoxin 500 mcg in 0.9% saline IV over 1 hour or 500 mcg orally at 12 hourly intervals for three doses, then 62.5–250 mcg daily
  - Beta-blocker e.g. metoprolol 25–100 mg tds orally
  - Verapamil 40–120 mg tds orally
  - Diltiazem 60–120 mg tds
  - Amiodarone is poorly effective at rapidly controlling rate in AF when given orally, but can be given as amiodarone 300 mg IV over 1 hour (then consider 1200 mg over 24 hours given centrally) and then/or 400 mg tds orally for 7 days. Amiodarone may result in cardioversion so should be avoided in inadequately anticoagulated patients
- Digoxin and amiodarone are the drugs of choice for patients with known structural heart disease and impaired left ventricular function
- Caution with combining diltiazem or verapamil with beta-blockers.

⑦ 3. Minimally symptomatic AF with no haemodynamic compromise

Ventricular rate <100 bpm, good perfusion.

Onset <48 hours
- Heparin (5–10,000 iu IV) then subcutaneous low-molecular weight
- In younger patients consider restoring sinus rhythm with amiodarone or flecainide where appropriate. A strategy to observe and wait for spontaneous cardioversion may also be adopted providing anticoagulation is initiated
- DC cardioversion can be considered within 48 hours of onset or electively after adequate anticoagulation.

Onset >48 hours
- Anticoagulation and rate control (if required) initially
- Antiarrhythmic therapy may be required to facilitate elective cardioversion once anticoagulated or to control excessive tachycardia during exertion.

Subsequent management
- Echocardiography to look for underlying heart disease
- Consider anticoagulation with warfarin, especially if structural heart disease, age >70, other risk factors for stroke, cardioversion performed when AF present for >48 hours, or if planning outpatient cardioversion in 4 weeks time
- Future antiarrhythmic strategy to prevent recurrence if previous episodes or presentation with compromising AF.

Special considerations for AF
- Rapid control of ventricular rate in the Emergency Room or ICU setting may also be achieved with a continuous infusion of the intravenous beta-blocker esmolol. This has the advantage of being short-acting and can be titrated up and down depending upon heart rate and blood pressure response
- Digoxin as a sole agent can slow the resting ventricular rate, but its effect may be lost once the patient becomes active and mobile.

⚙ Pre-excited atrial fibrillation
Pre-excited AF (p.331) conducted through an accessory pathway (a very rapid, irregular, broad complex tachycardia producing severe symptoms) should be treated with intravenous flecainide 2 mg/kg (max 150 mg) over 10–15 minutes. Flecainide slows conduction through both the AV node and accessory pathway. Avoid drugs that block AV node conduction (e.g. digoxin, verapamil, and adenosine). An alternative treatment for pre-excited AF is DC cardioversion.

Atrial flutter

- Atrial flutter is a macro-reentrant atrial tachycardia with an electrical wavefront that typically rotates around the tricuspid valve, although other, less common circuits may present as atypical flutters
- Like AF, atrial flutter may be paroxysmal, persistent, or permanent
- The typical atrial flutter circuit is restricted to the right atrium and the rest of the heart is activated passively
- The atrial rate is usually a regular 280–320 beats per minute, with the ventricles activated in a 2:1 fashion due to the filtering effect of the AV node
- Higher degrees of AV block may occur spontaneously or with the addition of drug therapy
- Rarely, 1:1 conduction may occur, leading to extremely rapid ventricular rates and severe symptoms
- Symptoms result from the rapid ventricular rate and loss of atrial contribution to ventricular filling and cardiac output. Patients may be asymptomatic, have palpitations, chest pain or dyspnoea, presyncope, syncope, or frank pulmonary oedema
- As with AF, the thromboembolic risk needs to be considered when considering the various treatment strategies.

Principle causes

Idiopathic, hypertension, mitral valve disease, cardiomyopathy (ischaemic, dilated or hypertrophic), acute infection, post-operative.

ECG diagnosis

Typical atrial flutter has a 'saw-tooth' baseline with flutter waves at 300 bpm with mainly negative deflections in leads II, III and aVF. When there is 2:1 conduction to the ventricle, flutter waves may be hard to see as alternate flutter waves are hidden in the QRS complex. The ventricular rate is usually regular at approximately 150 bpm. ECG 📖 p.332.

Treatment

Two strategies are available (as for AF)—either the restoration of sinus rhythm, or ventricular rate control. Some pharmacological treatments may address both. The treatment strategy should be based on haemodynamic compromise and thromboembolic risk.

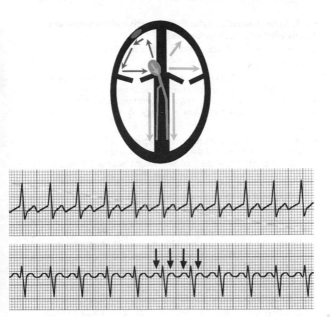

Atrial flutter. Regular QRS complexes, typically at 150 bpm. Rapid, regular atrial activity usually between 280 and 320 bpm (one flutter wave every large square). During 2:1 AV conduction alternate flutter waves may be hidden in QRS complexes. Lead V1 is often a good lead for spotting atrial activity (arrows). In typical flutter the flutter waves are negative in leads II, III and aVF (sawtooth pattern). Black arrows indicate a compulsory part of the rhythm/circuit, grey arrows indicate bystander (non-participating) pathways.

✿ 1. Atrial flutter with severe haemodynamic compromise

Ventricular rate >150 bpm or 1:1 conduction, hypotension and hypoperfusion, pulmonary oedema, cardiac ischaemia.

- Oxygen
- Heparin (5–10,000 iu IV) then subcutaneous low-molecular weight
- Synchronized DC shock under sedation/general anaesthesia using 200 J–360 J or equivalent biphasic energy.

① 2. Symptomatic atrial flutter with mild–moderate haemodynamic compromise

2:1 conduction, breathless and/or mild hypotension.

Onset <48 hours
- Heparin (5–10,000 iu IV) then subcutaneous low-molecular weight
- Pharmacological cardioversion with amiodarone 300 mg IV over 1 hour
- Synchronized DC shock under sedation/general anaesthesia
- 200 J–360 J or equivalent biphasic energy.

Onset >48 hours
- Subcutaneous low-molecular weight heparin
- Rate control with one of the following:
  - Digoxin 500 mcg in 0.9% saline IV over 1 hour or 500 mcg orally at 12 hourly intervals for three doses, then 62.5–250 mcg daily
  - Metoprolol 25–100 mg tds orally
  - Verapamil 40–120 mg tds orally
  - Diltiazem 60–120 mg tds
  - Amiodarone is poorly effective at rapidly controlling rate in atrial flutter when given orally but can be given as amiodarone 300 mg IV over 1 hour (then consider 1200 mg over 24 hours given centrally) and then/or 400 mg tds orally for 7 days. Amiodarone may result in cardioversion so should be avoided in inadequately anticoagulated patients
- Digoxin and amiodarone are the drugs of choice for patients with known structural heart disease and impaired left ventricular function. Amiodarone may however result in cardioversion back to sinus rhythm.

⑦ 3. Minimally symptomatic atrial flutter with no haemodynamic compromise

Ventricular rate <100 bpm, good perfusion.

Onset <48 hours
- Heparin (5–10,000 iu IV) then subcutaneous low-molecular weight
- Restore sinus rhythm as for AF with amiodarone or DC cardioversion
- A strategy to observe and wait for spontaneous cardioversion may also be adopted providing anticoagulation is started.

Onset >48 hours
- Consider anticoagulation
- Consider addition of antiarrhythmic to facilitate elective cardioversion once anticoagulated, or to improve rate control during exertion.

equent management
nocardiography to look for underlying heart disease
onsider anticoagulation with warfarin, especially if structural heart
disease, age >70, other risk factors for stroke, cardioversion performed
when flutter present for >48 hours, or if planning outpatient
cardioversion in 4 weeks time
• Consider future antiarrhythmic or radiofrequency ablation strategy to
prevent recurrence if this is not the first episode.

Special considerations for atrial flutter

▶ Flecainide should not be given to patients in atrial flutter without
additional AV nodal blocking drugs (e.g. beta-blockers).
• Flecainide and other Class 1C drugs may slow the flutter rate within
the atrium, allowing 1:1 conduction through the AV node and
a paradoxical increase in ventricular rate with worsening of symptoms
• Digoxin has less of an effect in atrial flutter that in AF
• Digoxin, verapamil, and adenosine should be avoided in AF or flutter
where there is also ventricular pre-excitation as they may increase
conduction through the accessory pathway.

Atrial tachycardia

- Sometimes called 'ectopic' or 'focal' atrial tachycardia and results fr
  a discrete focus firing automatically at a rate greater than the sinus
  node. Common sources of tachycardia are the pulmonary veins in the
  left atrium and the crista terminalis in the right atrium. The ventricle is
  often activated in a 1:1 fashion unless the atrial rate is particularly
  fast (>200 bpm) or AV nodal blocking drugs are being used
- Symptoms result from the rapid ventricular rate and usually manifest
  as palpitation, dyspnoea, presyncope or chest pain.

Principle causes

In children and young adults the heart is often structurally normal. In
older patients it is most likely to be associated with structural heart
disease. It may often occur in the setting of an acute illness or trauma
(sepsis, surgery, injury).

ECG diagnosis

Discrete P waves on the ECG, usually of a different shape to the P waves
present in sinus rhythm. Often has a normal PR interval with 1:1 or 2:1
conduction to ventricles. Often categorized as a 'long RP tachycardia'
(P to R wave shorter than R wave to next P wave). ECG 📖 p.333.

Treatment

Treatment should be addressed to any underlying cause (infection,
trauma etc).

☼ 1. Severe haemodynamic compromise

- Restore sinus rhythm with synchronized DC 200 J–360 J shock under
  sedation/general anaesthesia with anaesthetic support
- If the underlying cause is still present however, there is a high chance
  of recurrence. Start amiodarone (oral or IV).

① 2. Mild haemodynamic compromise

- Normal echo and/or no history of structural heart disease
  - Beta-blocker e.g. metoprolol 25–100 mg tds orally
  - Verapamil 40–120 mg tds orally
  - Amiodarone 300 mg over 1 hour IV then 400 mg tds orally
  - Flecainide 50–150 mg bd orally (use only after cardiology advice)
  - Digoxin 500 mcg in 0.9% saline IV over 1 hour or 500 mcg orally
    at 12 hourly intervals for three doses, then 62.5–250 mcg daily
- Sepsis, hypotension or structural heart disease
  - Beta-blocker e.g. metoprolol 25–100 mg tds orally (if structural
    heart disease but no hypotension or heart failure)
  - Amiodarone 300 mg over 1 hour IV then 400 mg tds orally
  - Digoxin 500 mcg in 0.9% saline IV over 1 hour or 500 mcg orally at
    12 hourly intervals for three doses, then 62.5–250 mcg daily.

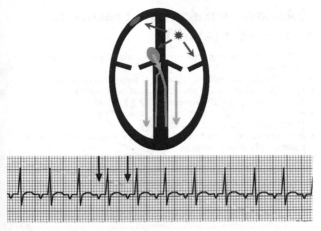

Atrial tachycardia. A focal, automatic tachycardia producing a discrete P wave, although the shape is usually different from the P wave shape seen during sinus rhythm. Usually 1:1 AV conduction unless a very rapid atrial rate or drugs have been given. May have subtle variations in heart rate. Black arrows indicate a compulsory part of the rhythm/circuit, grey arrows indicate bystander (non-participating) pathways.

① Atrioventricular nodal reentrant tachycardia (AVNRT)

- AVNRT is the commonest form of junctional reentrant tachycardia in adulthood
- The AV node is a critical component of the reentrant circuit
- It may present at any age and be sustained or non-sustained
- Heart rates are typically between 150 and 250 bpm
- In the typical form, the atria and ventricles are depolarized (and therefore contract) simultaneously
- Atrial contraction against closed AV valves can result in rapid, visible pulsation of the neck veins
- Usual symptoms are rapid palpitations with sudden onset and termination, dyspnoea, chest tightness, and pre-syncope
- AVNRT is most often seen in a structurally normal heart.

Principle causes

Attacks may be precipitated by exertion and physical or emotional stress, but are often spontaneous with no obvious cause.

ECG diagnosis

Usually narrow complex tachycardia, although may be broad complex if there is bundle branch block or rate-related aberrancy (typical RBBB or LBBB morphology will be present). Simultaneous atrial and ventricular depolarization means the P waves are usually hidden in the QRS and are not visible. In lead V1 the P wave may appear as a 'pseudo-R' wave at the end of the QRS complex. ECG 📖 p.334.

Treatment

- Tachycardia terminates if the AV node can be transiently blocked:
  - Vagal manoeuvres—carotid sinus massage, Valsalva manoeuvre, ocular pressure, ice application
  - Adenosine IV bolus (📖 p.136 for dose and administration)
- If tachycardia reinitiates immediately after adenosine administration, give verapamil 5–10 mg IV slow injection. Avoid if known impaired left ventricular function or significant hypotension as it may cause a further fall in blood pressure
- If 12 or 18 mg adenosine has no effect after being given appropriately, reconsider the diagnosis before giving verapamil
- DC cardioversion (200 J–360 J) if pharmacological treatment fails to terminate tachycardia.

Subsequent management

- With incessant tachycardia, start verapamil (initially 5–10 mg IV then 40–120 mg tds orally)
- Alternative drug treatments in the emergency setting include flecainide, esmolol or sotalol IV after consultation with a cardiologist
- First episodes do not usually require prophylactic drug therapy. Maintenance drug therapy or referral for radiofrequency ablation depends upon frequency, duration and severity of symptoms.

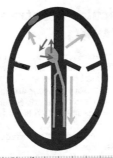

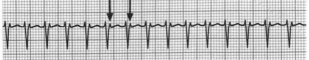

AV nodal reentrant tachycardia. A rapid, regular tachycardia. Usually narrow complex (unless bundle branch aberrancy occurs). Retrograde P wave occur during the QRS complex and are difficult to see, although typically appear as a 'pseudo-R wave' in lead V1 (arrows). Black arrows indicate a compulsory part of the rhythm/circuit, grey arrows indicate bystander (non-participating) pathways.

① Atrioventricular reentrant tachycardia (AVRT)

- AVRT is the result of an accessory pathway that connects the atria to the ventricles around the tricuspid or mitral valve annuli
- The AV node is also a critical component of the reentrant circuit
- Approximately $1/3^{rd}$ of accessory pathways are able to conduct antegradely from the atrium to the ventricles during sinus rhythm, producing ventricular pre-excitation (Wolff–Parkinson–White syndrome) ECG 📖 p.336.
- The remaining $2/3^{rds}$ can only conduct retrogradely from ventricles to atria (concealed accessory pathways)
- The usual form of tachycardia is conduction from atria to ventricles through the AV node and bundle branches (with normal ventricular depolarization) and conduction from the ventricles to the atria through the accessory pathway (orthodromic reciprocating tachycardia)
- Antidromic reciprocating tachycardia is much less common and results from antegrade conduction from the atria to the ventricles along the accessory pathway and retrograde conduction up through the AV node. Antidromic tachycardia can therefore only occur in those patients with ventricular pre-excitation
- Patients with Wolff–Parkinson–White syndrome have an increased risk of AF, which if conducted rapidly into the ventricles through the accessory pathway can lead to VF
- AVRT is usually seen in structurally normal hearts, although there is an association with Ebstein's anomaly and hypertrophic cardiomyopathy.

Principle causes and symptoms

- Attacks may be precipitated by exertion and physical or emotional stress, but are often spontaneous with no obvious cause
- Usual symptoms are rapid palpitations with sudden onset and termination, dyspnoea, chest tightness and pre-syncope or rarely syncope.

ECG diagnosis

Usually narrow complex tachycardia, although may be broad complex if there is bundle branch block or rate-related aberrancy (typical RBBB or LBBB morphology will be present). The retrograde P waves are often visible in the ST segment. ECG 📖 p.335.

Treatment

- As for AVNRT (📖 p.136)
- Pre-excited AF (📖 box p.143).

Subsequent management

- As for AVNRT (📖 p.136)
- In patients with ventricular pre-excitation (Wolff–Parkinson–White syndrome) avoid digoxin and verapamil maintenance therapy, particularly if there is a history of AF. Cardiology review is advised for risk stratification.

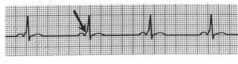

Sinus rhythm and pre-excitation. There is a short PR interval and delta wave at the beginning of the QRS (arrow). Black arrows indicate a compulsory part of the rhythm/circuit, grey arrows indicate bystander (non-participating) pathways.

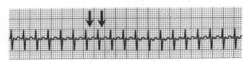

Orthodromic tachycardia. A rapid, regular rhythm. The circuit goes from atrium to ventricle through the AV node and bundle branches so the delta wave disappears and the QRS is narrow (unless there is bundle branch block aberrancy); then from ventricle to atrium through the accessory pathway. The retrograde P wave occurs after the QRS (arrows). Black arrows indicate a compulsory part of the rhythm/circuit, grey arrows indicate bystander (non-participating) pathways.

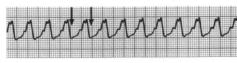

Antidromic tachycardia. Much less common. A rapid, regular rhythm. The circuit goes from atrium to ventricle through the accessory pathway so the ventricle is totally pre-excited and the QRS is very wide; then from ventricle to atrium through the bundle branches and AV node. The retrograde P wave occurs at the end of the QRS (arrows). Black arrows indicate a compulsory part of the rhythm/circuit, grey arrows indicate bystander (non-participating) pathways.

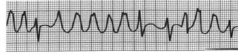

Pre-excited AF. AF is conducted to the ventricles through a combination of the AV node (narrow complexes) and the accessory pathway (wide, pre-excited complexes). The accessory pathway tends to dominate producing a very rapid ventricular rate. Black arrows indicate a compulsory part of the rhythm/circuit, grey arrows indicate bystander (non-participating) pathways.

☠ Ventricular fibrillation (VF)

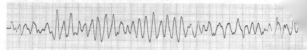

- Often a result of ischaemic heart disease (acute coronary syndrome, MI)
- Other cardiac precipitants include rapidly conducted AF via an accessory pathway (pre-excited AF p.143) and ion channelopathies (Brugada syndrome 📖 p.34)
- Needs immediate defibrillation (📖 p.302) using standard Advanced Life Support algorithms (📖 p.5)
- If VF is resistant to attempts at defibrillation then consider giving amiodarone 300mg IV and using a different defibrillator
- Treat reversible causes—correct K^+, Mg^{2+}
- Repeated episodes of VF (electrical storms) require specialist input (📖 p.162).

⚙️ Ventricular tachycardia (VT)

- VT is usually a reentrant arrhythmia that results from diseased or scarred myocardium
- Typically, patients have a history of ischaemic heart disease or non-ischaemic cardiomyopathy, although it may also occur in the setting of acute myocardial ischaemia or even the 'normal heart', where the mechanism may result from automaticity or triggered activity
- The ventricular rate may be anywhere between 100 and 300 bpm with symptoms ranging from none to palpitation, chest pain and dyspnoea, to haemodynamic collapse and cardiac arrest
- Tachycardia may be sustained or non-sustained
- The majority of episodes of VT are monomorphic i.e. the circuit is consistent and stable and the QRS morphology does not change
- Polymorphic VT results in a beat-to-beat variation in QRS morphology and in the setting of a prolonged corrected QT interval (QT^c) on the sinus rhythm ECG, is called 'torsade de pointes'
- Polymorphic VT usually causes collapse and is more often non-sustained although it may sustain and degenerate into VF.

⚙️ Monomorphic ventricular tachycardia

Principle causes

- Ischaemic heart disease (acute or chronic)
- Non-ischaemic cardiomyopathies (hypertrophic, dilated, arrhythmogenic right ventricular)
- Idiopathic (fascicular, verapamil-sensitive VT, right ventricular outflow tract VT).

ECG diagnosis

- Broad complex tachycardia (📖 p.136 for ECG diagnosis of broad complex tachycardia)
- Always make the diagnosis on a 12-lead ECG, not a rhythm strip
- Idiopathic varieties in normal hearts:
  - Fascicular VT typically has a QRS of 0.12–0.14 ms with RBBB and leftward axis morphology
  - Right ventricular outflow tract VT typically has a QRS of 0.12–0.15 ms with LBBB and inferior axis morphology.

Treatment

- VT that appears to be well tolerated has the potential to deteriorate rapidly so all treatments need to be instigated promptly, particularly in patients with known or suspected impairment of left ventricular function
- Only consider IV adenosine as a diagnostic or therapeutic manoeuvre if the arrhythmia is well tolerated or there is a high likelihood of SVT based on history or ECG.

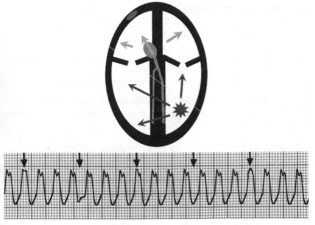

Monomorphic ventricular tachycardia. A regular, wide complex tachycardia. The QRS shape is constant although may be distorted by the independent P wave activity if there is visible AV dissociation (arrows). Black arrows indicate a compulsory part of the rhythm/circuit, grey arrows indicate bystander (non-participating) pathways.

1. VT with severe haemodynamic compromise

Reduced conscious level, pulmonary oedema, cardiac ischaemia, hypo
with poor perfusion.
- Oxygen
- Immediate synchronized DC shock under sedation/general anaesthesia
  (200 J–360 J or equivalent biphasic energy)
- Amiodarone 150 mg IV over 10 minutes through large vein.

2. VT with mild-moderate haemodynamic compromise

Hypotension with adequate perfusion, mild chest tightness or dyspnoea,
alert and orientated.
- Oxygen
- Inform anaesthetist and prepare for back-up DC cardioversion
- Amiodarone 150 mg IV over 10 minutes through large vein. May be
  repeated once. Monitor for hypotension
- If BP stable, consider lidocaine 50 mg IV over 2 minutes, repeated
  every 5 minutes until maximum of 200 mg
- If still VT, synchronized DC shock under sedation/general anaesthesia
  (200 J–360 J or equivalent biphasic energy).

Subsequent management of monomorphic VT
- Identify and treat underlying cause (ischaemia, MI)
- Check and replace electrolytes (potassium, magnesium)
- Recurrent episodes of VT require amiodarone or lidocaine infusions
  and possibly insertion of a temporary transvenous pacing wire for
  antitachycardia and overdrive pacing (📖 p.161)
- Consider giving magnesium sulphate (📖 p.160)
- Consider ongoing oral drug therapy with amiodarone and/or
  beta-blockers
- Seek urgent cardiology review (ICD therapy may be indicated).

☠ Polymorphic ventricular tachycar (‘Torsade de Pointes’)

Principal causes are:
- Congenital (long QT syndrome—ask about family history, deafness)
- Drugs (e.g. antiarrhythmics, macrolide antibiotics, tricyclic antidepressants)
- Electrolyte abnormalities (low K^+, low Mg^{2+}).

▶▶ Haemodynamic collapse is usually present or imminent if the arrhythmia is sustained. Urgent DC cardioversion is indicated.

▶ If conscious and stable, or polymorphic VT is repetitive and non-sustained:
- Check and correct electrolytes (K^+ Mg^{2+})
- If in sinus rhythm the QT^c interval is normal, Amiodarone 150 mg IV over 10 minutes through large vein. May be repeated once
- If the sinus rhythm QT^c is prolonged (>0.45 s) or unknown, give magnesium 1–2 mg in 100 mL 5% dextrose over 2–5 minutes, then 0.5–1 g/hr infusion
- If necessary, consider lidocaine 50 mg IV over 2 minutes, repeated every 5 minutes until maximum of 200 mg.

Subsequent management of polymorphic VT
- Identify and treat underlying cause (electrolytes, ischaemia, drugs)
- Potassium should be kept >4.0 mmol/L
- If there is a prolonged QT^c interval in sinus rhythm, especially in the setting of bradycardia, perform pacing with temporary transvenous pacing wire at 90–110 bpm
- Consider isoprenaline infusion (2–10 mcg/min prepared by diluting 1 mg in 500 mL of 5% Dextrose) as a temporary measure while awaiting pacing wire insertion
- If normal QT^c interval in sinus rhythm, give oral beta-blockers or amiodarone
- Seek urgent cardiology review.

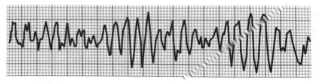

Torsade de Pointes. An irregular, broad complex tachycardia. The QRS axis twists around the baseline.

erdrive pacing

Sustained monomorphic VT may be terminated painlessly by anti-tachycardia pacing in 80–90% of cases

- After positioning a transvenous pacing wire in the right ventricle (☐ p.296), pacing is performed at a rate 15–20 bpm faster than the VT
- On many temporary pacing boxes there is a '× 3' setting on the rate for this reason
- A high output (5–10 V) may be required
- Capture of the VT is indicated by a change in QRS morphology and an increase in heart rate on the monitor to the pacing rate
- Pacing is abruptly terminated after 5–10 seconds of ventricular capture.

▶ There is a risk that acceleration of the VT may occur with degeneration to pulseless VT or VF so operators must be prepared for immediate defibrillation.

- Once sinus rhythm has been restored, constant background pacing at 90–110 bpm may be performed to prevent recurrent attacks. This is particularly useful with polymorphic VT and a prolonged QT interval, especially in the setting of pauses or bradycardia
- Constant ventricular pacing may result in decreased cardiac output due to the loss of AV synchrony, particularly in the setting of poor left ventricular function. This may be overcome with dual chamber AV sequential pacing.

✪ Electrical storms

▶ Seek early expert cardiology advice.

- VT or VF electrical storms are characterized by multiple, frequent, repetitive episodes of VT or VF
- Episodes may need to be terminated by repeated cardioversion or antitachycardia pacing
- Time, sedation with IV benzodiazepines, IV amiodarone and beta-blockade are the mainstays of treatment
- Correct the correctable (electrolytes, myocardial ischaemia, drug intoxication)
- Particular attention should be paid to potassium and magnesium levels
- IV amiodarone should be considered even if the patient has been on oral amiodarone therapy
- Alternative antiarrhythmic therapies include lidocaine or procainamide as an IV infusion (📖 p.166)
- Beta-blockers (e.g. esmolol, metoprolol) should be initiated as soon as possible
- In addition to pharmacological treatment and insertion of a temporary transvenous pacing wire for overdrive and antitachycardia pacing, patients often require intubation and ventilation to alleviate distress, increase oxygen delivery and reduce the hyperadrenergic state that may accompany repeated cardioversion
- If there is evidence of acute cardiac ischaemia, insertion of an intra-aortic balloon pump may increase coronary artery perfusion.

ⓘ **The ICD in the emergency room**

- Implantable cardioverter defibrillators (ICDs) are programmed to recognize ventricular rates that exceed programmed parameters. They are able to deliver antitachycardia pacing (which is painless) or shocks (which can be painful) within seconds of the tachycardia commencing
- It is common to program ICDs to attempt antitachycardia pacing for VT that is more likely to be haemodynamically tolerated, e.g. rates between 150 and 180 bpm. Shock therapy will only be delivered if antitachycardia pacing fails or the VT accelerates
- Very rapid VT or VF will often be treated by immediate shock therapy
- ICDs are able to deliver up to 6 shocks during a single VT or VF episode, however, if sinus rhythm is transiently restored the counter returns to zero and recommences if VT or VF reinitiates
- During VT or VF electrical storms, ICDs may deliver over 100 shocks within the space of a few hours
- Ventricular rates may also exceed programmed parameters and enter the detection zones in the setting of sinus tachycardia or atrial tachycardias
- Although ICDs try to distinguish between supraventricular tachycardia and VT, if the device is uncertain, it will always assume the worst and treat as if it is VT. Patients may therefore receive inappropriate shocks for sinus or atrial tachycardias with rapid ventricular rates.

One or two shocks

Patients who present to the emergency room having received one or two ICD shocks usually do not require hospital admission, particularly if this is not the first time. Providing they are otherwise well, they may be instructed to arrange a visit to their ICD clinic in the next 2–3 days to have device interrogation to check whether the shocks were appropriate.

Multiple shocks

If the patient has received multiple shocks over a short period of time, they require admission and assessment for electrolyte abnormalities or cardiac ischaemia, device interrogation and often an alteration in antiarrhythmic medication.

Use of a magnet

ICD shocks may be disabled by placing a magnet over the generator and securing with tape. This may be useful with repetitive inappropriate shocks due to device or lead failure or rapidly conducted atrial arrhythmias. It may also be appropriate as a temporary measure during electrical storms when VT is haemodynamically tolerated but resulting in frequent painful therapies.

▶ The patient must be monitored once a magnet is used as episodes of VF will not be treated by the ICD. The magnet does not disable the bradycardia functions of the ICD.

Commonly used antiarrhythmic agents in the emergency setting

Drug name	Dose

Amiodarone	• Cardiac arrest dose 300 mg as IV bolus
	• Slow IV bolus 150 mg over 10 mins
	  (in 100–250 mL 5% dextrose)
	• IV infusion to total 1.2 g in 500 mL 5% dextrose over
	  24 hours through central line
	• Oral 200–400 mg tds for 5–7 days then 200 mg
	  maintenance.

Digoxin	• IV loading 0.75–1 mg over 2 hours in 5% dextrose or 0.9% saline • Oral loading 1–1.5 mg 8 hourly over 24 hrs • Oral maintenance 62.5–250 mcg daily.

Esmolol	• Urgent IV bolus 1 mg/kg over 30 seconds
	• IV infusion 10 mg/mL in 5% dextrose or 0.9% saline.
	  Load with 0.5 mg/kg/min **for 1 minute only**.
	  Maintenance with 0.05–0.3 mg/kg/min, starting at
	  0.05 mg/kg/min.

Flecainide	• IV 2 mg/kg to a maximum of 150 mg over 15 minutes • Oral 50–150 mg twice daily.
Lidocaine	• IV bolus 50–100 mg over 1–2 minutes • Infusion 4 mg/minute for 30 minutes, 2 mg/minute for 2 hours, then 1 mg/minute.

Magnesium sulphate	• IV bolus 8 mmol (2 mg) over 5–10 minutes in 100 mL
	  5% dextrose
	• Infusion 2–4 mmol (0.5–1 g)/hr. Concentration should
	  not exceed 20%.

Procainamide	• IV 30 mg/min infusion up to a maximum total dose of 17 mg/kg • Maintenance infusion 1–4 mg/min.
Verapamil	• IV 5–10 mg over 2–3 minutes. Additional 5 mg after 5 minutes if necessary • Oral 40–120 mg tds.

Aortic dissection

Aortic dissection *170*
Marfan syndrome *176*
Acute thoracic syndromes *178*

☼ Aortic dissection

A tear in the aortic intima through which blood enters the aortic w
and strips the media from the adventitia.

- The dissection may result in fatal aortic rupture or propagate distally generating a blood-filled space between the dissected layers
- The blood supply to major branches (including the coronary arteries) may be compromised
- If the aortic root is involved, the aortic valve may become incompetent and retrograde propagation to the pericardium may result in cardiac tamponade.

The commonest site for aortic dissection is in the proximal ascending aorta within a few centimeters of the aortic valve or in the descending aorta just distal to the left subclavian artery.

Classification is usually made according to the Stanford classification that influences subsequent management:

☼ **Type A** aortic dissection involves the ascending aorta and management is a surgical emergency. Don't dawdle!

ⓘ **Type B** aortic dissection spares the ascending aorta and management is initially medical, with urgent blood pressure control and pain relief.

Causes and associations
- Hypertension (70%)
- Bicuspid aortic valve (7–14%) (📖 p.112)
- Marfan syndrome (5–9%) (📖 p.176)
- Aortic coarctation (📖 p.226)
- Iatrogenic (angiography).

Presentation
▶ The cardinal symptom is *pain* and is usually instantaneous, of cataclysmic severity, pulsatile or tearing, in the anterior thorax or interscapular region, and migrates as the dissection propagates.

Clinical signs
▶ There may be none.
- The patient may appear shocked but blood pressure can be normal or elevated
- Pulmonary oedema can occur due to severe aortic regurgitation
- Absent or reduced pulses occur in 20% of patients (but can fluctuate)
- Signs of aortic regurgitation or pericardial tamponade can occur in Type A aortic dissection
- A left pleural effusion is occasionally seen.

...tions

● ...normal aortic silhouette appears in up to 90% of cases.
...te, 10% of chest X-rays will appear normal)
...paration of the intimal calcification that occurs in the aortic knob
...by more than 1 cm (the 'calcium sign') is suggestive of aortic dissection
● Left sided pleural effusions can occur and are more common with
descending dissections.

ECG
● Non-specific ST and T wave changes are common
● ECG changes of left ventricular hypertrophy may occur in patients
with long-standing hypertension
● Coronary artery involvement is uncommon but more commonly
affects the right coronary artery (resulting in inferior ST elevation).

Blood tests
▶ May delay diagnosis so do not await results before arranging further
imaging.
● A mildly raised white cell count is common.

Imaging
Computed tomography
With modern spiral scanners, this has a sensitivity and specificity of
96–100% and is the standard investigation for suspected aortic dissection.

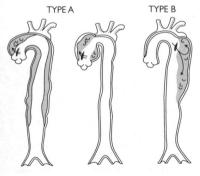

TYPE A   TYPE B

Stanford classification of aortic dissection. Type A: All dissections involving
the ascending aorta. Type B dissection does not involve the ascending aorta.

Magnetic resonance imaging
Sensitivity and specificity of nearly 100%. Non-invasive. Availabr
reduced access to an unwell patient are the main limitations on its t

Transoesophageal echocardiography
Useful for imaging the proximal ascending aorta, identifying involveme
of coronary ostia and examining the aortic valve. Sensitivity of ~98% an
specificity of ~95%. Patients usually require sedation. It is ideally performed immediately prior to surgery after surgical consent has been
obtained.

Transthoracic echocardiography
Can determine the involvement of the aortic valve, left ventricular function and identify pericardial effusions. Sensitivity of 59–85% and specificity
of 63–96%.

▶ A normal transthoracic echocardiogram does not exclude aortic
dissection.

Aortography
Invasive procedure with associated risks. Requires contrast material and
takes time to perform. Sensitivity of 77–88% and specificity of 94%. It is
now rarely performed as other imaging techniques are quicker and safer.

Coronary angiography
Not routinely performed in patients with aortic dissection. Chronic
coronary disease is seen in a quarter of patients with aortic dissection
but this has not been shown to have a significant impact on outcome.

Differential diagnosis
- Intramural haematoma 🕮 p. 178
- Penetrating atherosclerotic ulcer 🕮 p. 178
- Acute coronary syndrome 🕮 p. 46.

Pharmacological management
▶ Opiate analgesia should be given to eliminate pain.
▶ Lower systolic blood pressure to less than 120 mmHg with
  intravenous antihypertensive drugs:
  - Beta-blockers and the vasodilator sodium nitroprusside are the
    traditional first-line therapies (see box)
  - IV isosorbide dinitrate and oral nifedipine are alternatives in patients
    with contraindications to beta-blockers.
In hypotensive patients, it is important to exclude pericardial tamponade
and check the blood pressure in both arms before commencing fluid
resuscitation. ❶ Pericardiocentesis should not be performed prior to
surgery, as it can precipitate irretrievable haemodynamic collapse.

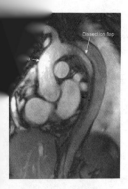

Magnetic resonance image of a **Type B** aortic dissection. There is a dissection flap in the descending aorta.

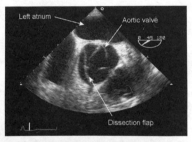

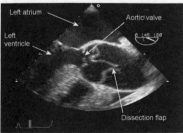

Transoesophageal echocardiography showing a **Type A** aortic dissection. Just above the aortic valve in the proximal ascending aorta is a dissection flap. Top: transverse view. Bottom: longitudinal view.

Intravenous antihypertensive therapy

- **Labetalol** is a beta-blocker with alpha-blocking effects at high do̤.
  It is given as an intravenous injection of 50 mg over 1 minute
  followed by a continuous infusion of 1–2 mg/min
- **Esmolol** is a short acting beta-blocker. It is administered as a bolus
  of 500 mcg/kg and as an infusion of 50–200 mcg/kg/min
- **Propranolol** is given as an intravenous injection of 1 mg over
  1 minute and repeated every 5 minutes until an adequate response
  has been achieved or a total of 10 mg has been given. Additional
  propranolol should then be given every 4 hours
- **Sodium nitroprusside** is given as an initial infusion of 0.5–
  1.5 mcg/kg/minute increasing in steps of 0.5 mcg/kg/minute every
  5 minutes. Dose range 0.5–8 mcg/kg/minute. It is usually given with
  a beta-blocker to prevent reflex tachycardia.

Surgical management

▶ *Type A* aortic dissection (involving the ascending aorta) should be considered for emergency surgery.

▶ *Type B* aortic dissections are usually managed medically. Surgery for type B dissections should be considered if there is evidence of proximal extension, progressive aortic enlargement or ischaemic complications from major branch artery involvement. Surgical risk is high.

Endovascular aortic stenting

Endovascular stenting is a percutaneous procedure that may be considered for aortic dissection starting distal to the left subclavian artery or to treat the complications of penetrating aortic ulcers.

Complications of aortic dissection
Type A
- Death from aortic rupture
- Myocardial ischaemia/infarction
- Pericardial tamponade
- Aortic valve incompetence
- Cerebrovascular event.

Type B
- Visceral ischaemia
- Limb ischaemia
- Renal failure.

...is

- ...nortality from aortic dissection is initially as high as 1% per hour
  surgical mortality is about 10–15% for type A dissection and
  ...ghtly higher for type B
- ...he long-term survival for patients with either surgically treated type A
  or medically treated type B dissections is about 75% at 5 years
- The false lumen commonly remains patent during long-term follow up.

Follow up

- Long-term oral antihypertensive therapy should be initiated to maintain
  a systolic blood pressure below 130 mmHg
- Drug therapies include beta-blockers, ACE-inhibitors, and calcium
  antagonists
- Surveillance is recommended for all patients using the imaging modality
  with which there is the most local expertise, particularly in the first
  two years after presentation
- Surgery or endovascular stenting should be considered if there is
  evidence of progressive aortic enlargement.

References

Nienaber CA and Eagle KA (2003). Aortic dissection: new frontiers in diagnosis and management.
  Part I: from etiology to diagnostic strategies. *Circulation* **108**, 628–635.
Nienaber CA and Eagle KA (2003). Aortic dissection: new frontiers in diagnosis and management.
  Part II: therapeutic management and follow-up. *Circulation* **108**, 772–778.

Marfan syndrome

- Autosomal dominant connective tissue disease with a prevalence of at least 1:10,000
- Common cardiovascular features are:
  - mitral valve prolapse (75%)
  - dilatation of the aortic sinuses (90%)
- Aortic dilatation is usually limited to the proximal ascending aorta with loss of the sinotubular junction and a flask shape appearance
- Aortic regurgitation is common when the aorta reaches 50 mm in diameter (normal diameter <40 mm)
- The risk of dissection increases with the diameter of the aorta but occurs relatively infrequently below a diameter of 55 mm
- Aortic dissection in Marfan syndrome is usually Type A and begins just above the coronary ostia. 10% of cases begin distal to the left subclavian artery (Type B)
- Beta blockade has been shown to reduce the rate of aortic dilatation and reduce the risk of aortic dissection
- Surgery is usually considered when the aorta reaches >50 mm.

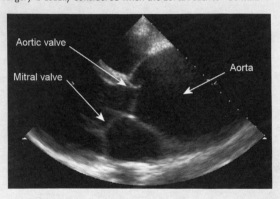

Transthoracic echocardiography of an enlarged ascending aorta in a patient with Marfan syndrome.

Weblink

- The Marfan Foundation *http://www.marfan.org*

Acute thoracic syndromes

☼ Intramural haematoma

- The result of haemorrhage within the media and adventitia of the aortic wall. The aortic intima remains intact
- Believed to be due to rupture of the aortic vasa vasorum
- Presentation can mimic aortic dissection
- Patients are typically elderly, with a history of hypertension and many have aortic atherosclerosis
- The diagnosis is made by excluding an intimal tear
- Computed tomography or magnetic resonance imaging are the investigations of choice. A non-contrast-enhancing crescent along the aortic wall with no false lumen or associated atherosclerotic ulcer is usually demonstrated
- There is increasing evidence that an intramural haematoma may be a precursor of aortic dissection
- Treat as for aortic dissection with analgesia and IV anti-hypertensive agents
- Surgery is indicated when the ascending aorta is involved.

① Penetrating atherosclerotic ulcer

- Ulceration of an atherosclerotic lesion of the aorta that penetrates the elastic lamina of the aorta allowing haematoma formation within the media
- Usually in the descending aorta in elderly smokers
- Clinical presentation is similar to aortic dissection with chest or back pain
- In up to 25% of cases, penetration through to the adventitia results in false aneurysm formation and transmural aortic rupture occurs in up to 10% of cases
- Aortography is the diagnostic standard
- Standard treatment is high risk surgery but there has been increasing success with the use of endovascular stenting.

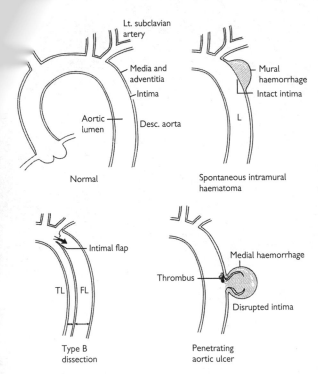

Acute thoracic syndromes. An intramural haematoma is characterized by an intact intima. Type B aortic dissection usually starts distal to the left subclavian artery. A penetrating aortic ulcer involves a disrupted intima and haemorrhage into the media.

Chapter 11

Pericardial disease

Pericarditis *182*
Pericardial tamponade *184*
Constrictive pericarditis *186*

⑦ Pericarditis

Inflammation of the pericardium—may involve adjacent myocardium ('peri-myocarditis').

Causes

- Often idiopathic
- Viral (e.g. Coxsackie, Epstein–Barr)—history of recent mild generalized illness is not uncommon but specific virus rarely identified
- Bacterial—tuberculous, acute rheumatic fever, pneumonia
- Uraemia
- Autoimmune (systemic lupus erythematosus, rheumatoid arthritis)
- Post-MI—2 time periods:
  - Acute—few days post MI, esp. if large
  - Later—2–8 weeks (as part of Dressler syndrome 📖 p.60)
- Post-cardiac surgery
- Hypothyroidism
- Chest radiotherapy
- Trauma (e.g. blunt chest injury 📖 p.280).

Presentation

- Chest pain (📖 p.16 for differential diagnosis)
  - Typically retrosternal soreness/ache; can be sharp
  - Sometimes positional (worse on lying flat when visceral and parietal pericardium rub together; better sitting up)
  - ± Radiation to shoulder/scapula/back
  - Can be worse with deep inspiration
  - Onset over hours, occasionally minutes/sudden
- ± SOB (usually mild)
- May be history of coryzal illness in preceding 1–3 weeks.

Clinical signs

- Often none
- Pericardial rub—rough sound 'like feet crunching on snow' or 'saw-like' in both systole & diastole, best heard at the left sternal edge. Similar to pleural rub, but synchronized to cardiac cycle. *Clinches the diagnosis!*
- Rarely, signs of tamponade may be present (📖 p.184).

Investigations

- ECG (can be normal in 10%)—two main patterns:
    1. 'Scooped' or 'saddle-shaped' ST elevation in several leads; may not correspond to coronary artery distribution (📖 p.323)
    2. Non-specific T-wave inversion
  - Look for PR segment depression. It is highly specific for pericarditis
- Blood tests—FBC, CRP, blood cultures (?infection), U&E (?uraemia), thyroid function (?hypothyroid), ASO titre (?rheumatic fever), ± autoimmune screen
- Cardiac troponins—may be raised in pericarditis; more common if ST elevation on ECG and probably represents perimyocarditis
- An echocardiogram should be considered in patients with pericarditis who are systemically unwell and/or hypotensive (?pericardial effusion, ?myocarditis). It can also be useful to exclude acute MI in difficult cases (MI: regional left ventricular dysfunction corresponding to coronary artery territory)
- If a pericardial effusion is confirmed then pericardial fluid can be sent for Ziehl–Nielsen staining, cytology, protein, LDH (📖 p.300 for peri-cardiocentesis).

Diagnostic clues

- History, especially the character of pain
- Patient often younger and usually relatively well compared to typical MI patient, not clammy/grey/sweaty
- The ECG can sometimes look like an acute MI but does not have reciprocal changes, and the history and well appearance of the patient are usually clues against this. The correct diagnosis is important, as giving thrombolysis to a patient with pericarditis can risk haemorrhagic tamponade. If in real doubt, an echocardiogram can be helpful.

❶ Cardiac troponins are not a discriminator between MI and pericarditis (troponin I can be elevated to double figures).

Management

- Analgesia—NSAIDs/aspirin often very effective (e.g. diclofenac 50 mg TDS po or ibuprofen 400 mg TDS po). Others include paracetamol ± codeine (e.g. co-dydramol 500/30 2 tabs QDS), colchicine 500 mg BD po (for recurrent attacks), steroids or immunosuppressants for resistant recurrent episodes
- Treat any identified cause
- Observe for tamponade if large pericardial effusion present—drain if necessary
- Uncomplicated cases do not need hospital admission.

:☼: Pericardial tamponade

Causes

- As per pericarditis (📖 p.182)
- May occur as a complication of percutaneous coronary intervention and electrophysiology procedures—be aware in the hypotensive patient just returned to the ward
- Large effusions are commonly associated with malignancy, uraemia, or tuberculosis
- Tamponade without inflammatory signs (pain, friction rub, fever, diffuse ST elevation) is usually associated with a malignant effusion.

Presentation

- Chest discomfort (as per pericarditis)
- Breathlessness
- Faintness and syncope
- Cough and dysphagia
- With signs of its complications (renal failure, hepatic ischaemia, etc.).

Clinical signs

- Tachycardia is almost universal (>100 beats/min)—may be lower in hypothyroid and uraemia
- Reduced pulse pressure
- Hypotension (may be normal in pre-existing hypertension)
- Jugular venous distension (rises on inspiration—Kussmaul's sign)
- Pulsus paradoxus (the normal systolic pressure difference between inspiration and expiration is increased to over 10 mmHg. Clinically the pulse fades on inspiration)
- Muffled heart sounds, non-palpable apex beat
- Dyspnoea or tachypnoea with clear lungs.

Investigations

- ECG—reduced voltages, changing axis (as the heart swings in the fluid)
- CXR—globular heart, convex or straight left heart border
- Transthoracic echocardiography—common findings include:
  - Pericardial effusion (📖 p.185)
  - Diastolic collapse of right ventricular free wall and right atrium
  - Dilated inferior vena cava with no inspiratory collapse and reversed flow with atrial contraction
  - Tricuspid flow increases during inspiration
  - Mitral flow decreases during inspiration.

Management

- Pericardiocentesis should be performed urgently (📖 p.300)—removing only a small amount of fluid can improve haemodynamics considerably
- Medical management includes fluid resuscitation (but should not delay definitive treatment).

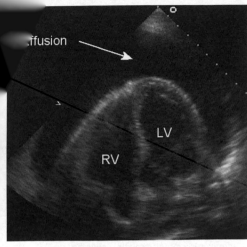

Transthoracic echocardiography demonstrating a large pericardial effusion over-lying the left (LV) and right (RV) ventricles.

① Constrictive pericarditis

Imprisons the heart. Resembles congestive cardiac failure but the c
picture is not due to heart 'failure', rather the cardiac function has b
impeded due to impaired filling.

Causes
- Most cases are idiopathic—the initial acute episode may be subclinical
- Viral, tuberculous and pyogenic infections
- Therapeutic irradiation
- Post cardiac surgery.

Presentation and signs
- Chronic venous congestion with prominent *x* and *y* descents in the JVP
- Oedema
- Hypotension
- Abdominal distension—ascites, hepatosplenomegaly
- Loud or palpable S_3 due to rapid ventricular filling (pericardial knock)
- Atrial arrhythmias are common.

Investigations
- Exclude TB—Mantoux, early morning sputum and urine
- ECG—Non-specific T wave abnormalities with low voltages, broad
  P wave, AF
- CXR—pericardial calcification (lateral films), pleural effusions
- Echocardiography—findings include:
  - Pericardial thickening and calcification with biatrial enlargement
  - Rapid early filling (increased E:A ratio)
  - Dilated venae cavae and hepatic veins with restricted
    respiratory fluctuations
  - Paradoxical ventricular septal movement with a flat posterior wall
  - Increased tricuspid flow and reduced mitral flow in inspiration
    (similar to tamponade)
- CT/MRI—Pericardial thickening (>6 mm) and calcification, biatrial
  enlargement, dilated venae cavae and hepatic veins
- Cardiac catheterization—useful to differentiate from restrictive
  cardiomyopathy (📖 p.82) and to exclude co-existent coronary
  artery disease. Typical findings are:
  - Left ventricular end diastolic pressure = right ventricular end
    diastolic pressure throughout respiration (different by >7 mmHg in
    restrictive cardiomyopathy). Both are elevated and have a dip and
    plateau (square root) configuration
  - Atrial pressures are high and equal with prominent *x* and *y*
    descents.

Management
- Diuretic therapy, salt restriction
- Surgical pericardectomy is usually required
- Balloon dilatation of the pericardium can be considered as a palliative
  procedure.

Pulmonary vascular disease

Pulmonary embolism 190
Pulmonary hypertension 196

① Pulmonary embolism

The annual incidence of pulmonary embolism (PE) is 60–70/100,0▢ half of cases occurring in hospital. In hospital mortality ranges 6–15%. The most common cause is venous thromboembolism (V▢ but non-thrombotic causes include air, fat, amniotic fluid, and tum▢ fragments.

The diagnosis of PE should be based on a combination of clinical assessment and appropriate imaging.

Presentation and signs

- Most patients with PE are breathless (82% of cases) and/or tachypnoeic (respiratory rate >20/min, 60% of cases)
- Patients may also present with chest pain (49% of cases), cough, syncope and haemoptysis
- Tachycardia and fever are common
- Elevated JVP, loud P_2, hypotension, gallop rhythm, pleural rub, cyanosis may occur.

Patients should be clinically assessed into low, intermediate, and high clinical probability of PE.

Clinical probability

- The patient must have clinical features of PE: breathlessness and/or tachypnoea with or without chest pain and/or haemoptysis
- Two other clinical factors are sought:
  - (a) The absence of another reasonable clinical explanation and
  - (b) The presence of a major risk factor
- Where (a) and (b) are true the probability is *high*
- If only one is true the probability is *intermediate*
- If neither is true the probability is *low*.

✺ Massive PE

Massive PE is highly likely if *all* the features below are present:

- Collapse/hypotension
- Unexplained hypoxia
- Engorged neck veins
- Right ventricular gallop.

risk factors

or abdominal/pelvic surgery
cent hip/knee replacement
Lower limb fracture
Varicose veins
- Recent caesarian section
- Post-partum period
- Abdominal/pelvic malignancy
- Advanced/metastatic malignancy
- Prolonged hospitalization/institutional care
- Previous venous thromboembolism.

Minor risk factors

- Congestive cardiac failure
- Congenital heart disease
- Hypertension
- Superficial venous thrombosis
- In-dwelling central venous catheter
- Oral contraceptive pill
- Hormone replacement therapy
- COPD
- Thrombotic disorders
- Long distance sedentary travel.

Investigations

Blood tests
- Arterial blood gases (hypoxaemia)
- FBC, U&E, D-dimer (see below)
- Cardiac troponin may be elevated due to right heart strain but is not of diagnostic value.

D-dimer assay
- Should only be performed following assessment of clinical probability
- Need not be performed in those with a high clinical probability of PE
- A negative assay reliably excludes PE in patients with low or intermediate clinical probability.

Thrombophilia screen
Testing for thrombophilia should be considered in patients aged under 50 with recurrent PE or in those with a strong family history of proven VTE.

ECG
- Most common finding is sinus tachycardia
- Non-specific ST and T wave changes are common
- Incomplete or complete right bundle branch block and right ventricular strain pattern occur. The classic $S_1Q_3T_3$ pattern is rare (ECG opposite).

CXR
- Used to exclude conditions that mimic PE (chest infection, pneumothorax)
- May show wedge-shaped peripheral infarcts or pulmonary effusions.

Other imaging
- CT pulmonary angiography (CTPA) is the recommended imaging tool
- Isotope lung scanning may be considered following a normal CXR if good quality facilities and reporting are on site and the patient has no significant concurrent cardiopulmonary disease. A non-diagnostic isotope lung scan should be followed by further imaging. There is also a high false positive rate. If isotope lung scanning is normal then PE is reliably excluded
- Venous ultrasonography. In patients with co-existing deep vein thrombosis, leg ultrasound is often sufficient to confirm VTE. A single normal leg ultrasound does not exclude subclinical DVT however
- Conventional pulmonary angiography can be considered in selected cases on advice from a cardiologist or radiologist (📖 p.195).

Echocardiography
- Can be abnormal in massive PE (right heart dilatation) and can provide non-invasive information on pulmonary artery pressures
- May provide an alternative diagnosis (aortic dissection, pericardial tamponade, myocardial dysfunction)
- There is little additional benefit from trans-oesophageal echocardiography.

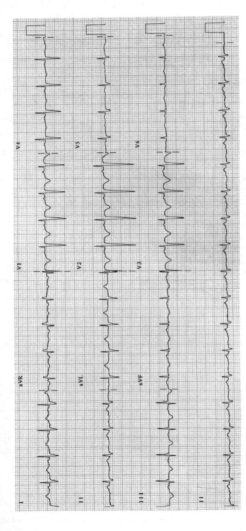

ECG in massive PE. Sinus tachycardia with widespread T wave inversion. There is a large S wave in V1 with a Q wave and T inversion in lead III.

Management
- Institute resuscitation measures according to haemodynamic status
  - Oxygen
  - Analgesia (opiates or NSAIDs if pleuritic pain)
  - Cautious volume expanders if hypotensive
  - Dobutamine for right-side heart failure and shock
- Heparin (usually low molecular weight) should be commenced before imaging if clinical probability of PE is low or intermediate
- Use unfractionated heparin when rapid reversal of anticoagulation is considered or in patients with massive PE when thrombolysis/invasive intervention is considered
- Oral anticoagulation should be started once VTE is confirmed, target INR is 2–3
- Current recommendations for duration of anticoagulation are: 4–6 weeks for temporary risk factors, 3 months for first idiopathic PE, at least 6 months for other causes.

Thrombolysis
- Evidence for reduction in mortality is sparse and thrombolysis should not be used as first line treatment in non-massive PE
- In patients with massive, life-threatening PE, give alteplase (rt-PA) 50 mg bolus
- In stable patients with confirmed massive PE, dose of rt-PA for thrombolysis is 100 mg over 90 minutes
- Should be followed by unfractionated heparin as an infusion
- Invasive approaches as an alternative or adjunct to thrombolysis (thrombus fragmentation or thrombectomy) should be considered on advice from a cardiologist or radiologist.

Reference

British Thoracic Society guidelines for the management of suspected acute pulmonary embolism. (2003). *Thorax* **58**, 470–484.

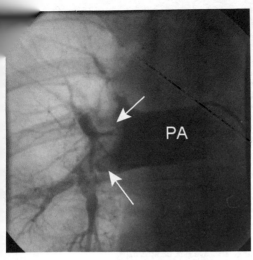

Pulmonary angiography of the right pulmonary artery (PA) demonstrating large filling defects (arrowed) in keeping with massive pulmonary emboli.

⑦ Pulmonary hypertension

- An increase in mean pulmonary arterial pressure >25 mmHg at rest >30 mmHg with exercise
- Classified by the World Health Organization according to common pathobiological features (see box opposite)
- Primary pulmonary hypertension is the diagnosis in patients with pulmonary arterial hypertension of unexplained aetiology
- Is usually already established when the patient presents.

Presentation

- Breathlessness is the usual complaint although some patients present with exertional syncope (fixed or reduced cardiac output) or angina (from right ventricular ischaemia)
- Patients with pulmonary venous hypertension relating to left heart disease will often have symptoms of orthopnoea and paroxysmal nocturnal dyspnoea
- Signs include:
  - Elevated JVP with a large a wave (large v wave if severe tricuspid regurgitation)
  - Low volume pulse
  - Right ventricular heave (left parasternal)
  - Loud pulmonary component of the second heart sound
  - Systolic murmur (tricuspid regurgitation)
  - Central and peripheral cyanosis
  - Oedema
  - Ascites
  - Signs of associated disease (e.g. sclerodactyly in scleroderma).

Investigations

- **ECG:** Right ventricular hypertrophy (📖 p.199) is highly specific but has a low sensitivity. Right bundle branch block with anterior ST abnormalities can occur. Prominent P waves (P pulmonale) suggest right atrial enlargement
- **CXR:** Enlargement of the pulmonary artery and its major branches. Tapering of peripheral arteries. Enlarged right atrium and ventricle
- **Bloods:** FBC, U&E, LFTs, ESR, arterial blood gases, thrombophilia screen, autoimmune profile
- **Echocardiography:** Enlarged right ventricle with septal flattening. Doppler estimate of pulmonary artery systolic pressure
- **Further specialist investigations include:**
  - High resolution CT scan
  - Lung perfusion scintigraphy
  - Pulmonary function tests (particularly gas transfer)
  - Hepatitis and HIV serology and viral titres
  - Exercise testing
  - Nocturnal oxygen saturation studies
  - Cardiac catheterization and pulmonary angiography after specialist advice (increased risk).

sification and causes

Pulmonary arterial hypertension
- Primary pulmonary hypertension (sporadic/familial)
- Associated with connective tissue disease, portal hypertension, HIV, drugs/toxins, other
- Pulmonary venous hypertension
  - Left-sided atrial or ventricular heart disease
  - Left-sided valvular disease
  - Extrinsic compression of central pulmonary veins
- Pulmonary hypertension associated with respiratory disease/hypoxaemia
  - Chronic obstructive pulmonary disease
  - Interstitial lung disease
  - Sleep disordered breathing
  - Alveolar hypoventilation disorders
  - Chronic exposure to high altitude
- Pulmonary hypertension due to chronic thrombotic/embolic disease
  - Thromboembolic obstruction of proximal pulmonary arteries
  - Obstruction of distal pulmonary arteries (PE, in situ thrombosis, sickle cell)
- Pulmonary hypertension due to pulmonary vascular disorders
  - Inflammatory (schistosomiasis, sarcoidosis, other)
  - Pulmonary capillary haemangiomatosis.

Management

- Making the initial diagnosis of pulmonary hypertension is important, but the actual cause may be difficult to identify quickly and is made after appropriate advice and investigation
- The management of patients presenting *de novo* with pulmonary hypertension includes appropriate use of oxygen to correct hypoxaemia, anticoagulation, and diuretic therapy
- Get specialist advice for patients known to have pulmonary hypertension who present unwell
- Long-term management includes:
  - Lifestyle changes (graded exercise activities)
  - Anticoagulation with warfarin (INR 2.5)
  - Diuretics (often high doses of loop diuretics are needed)
  - Supplemental oxygen therapy
- Therapies according to the underlying cause include:
  - Vasodilator therapy (<10% of patients benefit, see box)—high dose calcium channel blockers such as nifedipine (up to 240 mg/day) and diltiazem (up to 700 mg/day) are used
  - Prostacyclins—continuous infusion of epoprostenol
  - Endothelin receptor blockers—e.g. bosentan 125 mg BD
  - Phosphodiesterase inhibitors—e.g. sildenafil, tadalafil
  - Digoxin (to improve right ventricular function)
  - Atrial septostomy
  - Pulmonary thromboendarterectomy
  - Heart–lung and lung transplantation.

Vasodilator therapy in primary pulmonary hypertension

During right heart cardiac catheterization, pulmonary haemodynamics are measured. Short-acting vasodilator therapy is used (inhaled nitric oxide, nebulized prostacyclin or intravenous adenosine). A positive response is defined as a >20% reduction in mean pulmonary artery pressure or pulmonary vascular resistance without a decrease in cardiac output. Patients who respond and who have a cardiac index >2.1 L/min/m^2, and/or mixed venous oxygen saturation >63% and/or right atrial pressure <10 mmHg should be considered for calcium channel blockers.

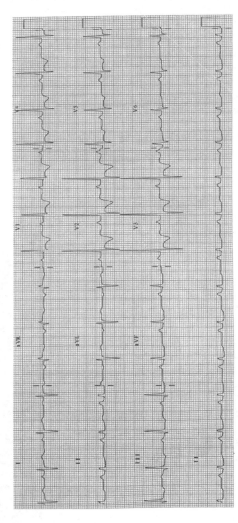

ECG in chronic severe pulmonary hypertension. Right ventricular hypertrophy is demonstrated by right axis deviation, large R waves with T wave inversion in leads V1–3 and a prominent p wave (p pulmonale).

Systemic emboli

Systemic emboli 202
Paradoxical emboli 204

! Systemic emboli

Embolization of material, usually thrombus or vegetation, leading to signs and symptoms of obstruction of a coronary, cerebral, or peripheral artery.

Presentation
- Transient ischaemic attack/stroke (common)
- Acute ischaemia of a limb (painful, pulseless, pale, paralysis)
- MI or acute coronary syndrome
- Acute small bowel ischaemia (superior mesenteric artery embolism)—abdominal pain, hypovolaemia, few abdominal signs
- Acute renal failure (rare).

Investigations
▶ **Should be guided by history and examination**
- FBC (anaemia, platelet count/clumping), U&Es
- ESR and D-dimer
- Coagulation screen
- ECG (AF, MI)
- CXR (cardiomegaly)
- CT head if stroke (to exclude haemorrhage, intracranial mass)
- Carotid/peripheral artery Doppler ultrasound
- Doppler ultrasound of leg veins (DVT)
- Echocardiography (📖 p.203).

Management
- Management of the presenting condition may be necessary before considering investigation for the source of embolism e.g. acute limb ischaemia, small bowel ischaemia
- Patients should be systemically anticoagulated if a cardiac source of embolism is demonstrated
- The use of early anticoagulation in embolic stroke is controversial and should be according to local policy
- PFO/ASD—device closure or surgery if appropriate
- DVT and PFO with contraindications to warfarin—consider device closure of PFO and inferior vena cava filter.

...ses

Carotid atheroma (common)
- Left atrial appendage thrombus
  - AF
  - Mitral stenosis
  - Impaired atrial function
- Left ventricular thrombus (post infarct, cardiomyopathy, left ventricular aneurysm, non-compaction)
- Left heart valves
  - Prosthetic (endocarditis, thrombosis)
  - Native (aortic stenosis, mitral stenosis)
- Cardiac shunt with paradoxical embolism
  - Atrial septal defect (ASD)
  - Patent foramen ovale (PFO)
  - Ventricular septal defect (with raised right ventricular pressure)
- Aorta
  - Atheroma
  - Dissection (📖 p.170)
- Cardiac tumours 📖 p.282
  - Myxoma
  - Other primary and secondary tumours (rare).

Echocardiography for systemic emboli

Indications for transthoracic echocardiography (TTE)
- Unexplained systemic embolism
- TTE is also indicated if clinical signs of endocarditis (📖 p.99), myxoma (📖 p.282)
▶ In the absence of a cardiac history, ECG abnormalities or clinical signs, TTE is unlikely to be useful.

Indications for transoesophageal echocardiography (TOE)
- Non-diagnostic TTE
- Endocarditis suspected and not confirmed on TTE
- Suspected prosthetic valve dysfunction
- Suspected PFO or ASD.

① Paradoxical emboli

Systemic embolism from the venous system crossing an abnormal communication within the heart (usually via an ASD or PFO).

- A PFO is the commonest cardiac abnormality found in young patients with unexplained stroke
- For a PFO to cause a systemic emboli the following triad is required:
  - The presence of the PFO
  - Raised right atrial pressure (permanent or transient e.g. coughing, straining)
  - Venous source of thrombosis (usually a deep vein thrombosis).

Saline contrast echocardiography

- Assesses right to left shunting using the Valsalva manoeuvre to increase right atrial pressure. In a normal study no bubbles should cross to the left heart
- If TTE positive, a TOE is still required to assess the atrial septum for suitability of device closure
- False negatives may occur: on TTE due to poor image quality; with TOE due to poor Valsalva manoeuvre and failure to increase right atrial pressure
- Injecting saline contrast via the femoral vein increases the diagnostic accuracy (blood is directed via the Eustachian valve towards the PFO).

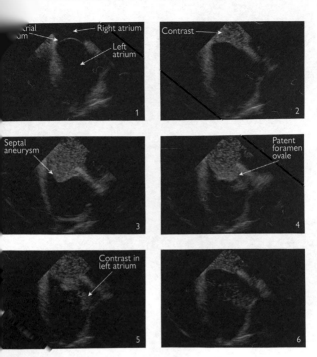

Intracardiac echocardiography study demonstrating passage of agitated saline contrast from the right atrium through a patent foramen ovale into the left atrium. The interatrial septum is aneurysmal.

Cardiac issues in pregnancy

Introduction *208*
Heart failure in pregnancy *210*
Aortic disease in pregnancy *210*
Acute MI in pregnancy *211*
Pulmonary embolism in pregnancy *211*
Valvular heart disease in pregnancy *212*
Arrhythmias in pregnancy *213*
Hypertension in pregnancy *214*
Anticoagulation in pregnancy *214*

Introduction

For patients with known cardiac disease, pregnancy should ideally be planned and undertaken following consideration of risks to the mother and fetus. In some cases it may be necessary to alter or stop treatment prior to conception (e.g. warfarin, ACE inhibitors).

Pregnancy may be associated with new presentations of heart disease. Be aware that pregnancy can:
• Unmask pre-existing conditions
• Exacerbate pre-existing conditions
• Precipitate new conditions.

Death during pregnancy is rare (approximately 1 per 50,000 pregnancies) but cardiac disease is the most common cause (e.g. cardiomyopathy, aortic dissection, myocardial infarction, complications of pulmonary hypertension).

Normal physiological changes in pregnancy

One of the challenges to diagnosing pregnancy-related heart disease is to distinguish pathological features from adaptive changes in cardiovascular function. Circulating volume, heart rate, stroke volume, and consequently cardiac output increase markedly in the first 16 weeks, plateau and then increase further in the weeks before term.

The following are all consistent with normal pregnancy:
• Fatigue
• Shortness of breath
• Palpitation, re-entrant SVT
• Atrial and ventricular premature beats
• Raised jugular venous pressure
• Pedal oedema
• Sinus tachycardia ~100 bpm
• Full volume, collapsing pulse
• 3rd heart sound
• Systolic flow murmur.

Clinical indicators of pathological states

• Chest pain
• Severe dyspnoea
• Orthopnoea, paroxysmal nocturnal dyspnoea
• Sinus tachycardia >100 at rest
• AF/atrial flutter
• Ventricular tachycardia
• Hypotension
• Pulmonary oedema
• Pleural effusion.

General principles of cardiac management

Avoid drugs if possible, and use the fewest drugs in the smallest doses BUT do not deny appropriate management because of pregnancy.

▶ Remember, if the mother is compromised, so is the fetus.
▶ Obtain EARLY advice from:
  • 'High-risk' obstetrician
  • Specialist cardiologist.

Heart failure in pregnancy

This accounts for 25% of all cardiac deaths in pregnancy. Mortality is up to 10% where left ventricular ejection fraction is ≤20%. Consider termination if heart failure occurs early in pregnancy.

Causes
- Dilated cardiomyopathy
- Underlying structural conditions e.g. valvular disease
- Peripartum cardiomyopathy is clinically indistinguishable from other dilated cardiomyopathies but, by definition, occurs only in the last month of pregnancy or up to 6 months post partum, *in the absence of any other cardiac pathology*. LV dysfunction persists in 50% and there is a significant risk of recurrence in subsequent pregnancies even when LV function has initially returned to normal. If LV function does not return to normal, the risk of death in any subsequent pregnancy is ~20%.

Acute management
- Similar to other forms of heart failure: bed rest
- Diuretics
- ⚠ ACE inhibitors contraindicated until delivery (risk of renal agenesis)
- Vasodilators: hydralazine is recommended in pregnancy.

Aortic disease in pregnancy

The major concern is aortic dissection which is usually associated with underlying aortic disease.

Causes and associations
- Marfan syndrome, especially with aortic root >4 cm (📖 p.176)
- Turner's syndrome (assisted conception) or mosaic Turner's ~2% risk of dissection in pregnancy
- Aortic coarctation (whether corrected or not)
- Bicuspid aortic valve with dilated aortic root. The risk of dissection in pregnancy is only slightly higher than in the general population.

General management
Patients at risk should have pre-conception evaluation of the aorta with echocardiography and/or magnetic resonance. In pregnancy, further monitoring is warranted. Beta-blockers through pregnancy are advised to reduce the risk of root dilation. If evidence of aortic dilatation, caesarian section should be undertaken to minimize haemodynamic stresses.

☼ Acute aortic dissection in pregnancy
▶ 📖 p.170 for general management.
- Pelvic wedge during supine imaging to prevent IVC obstruction
- Blood pressure control with beta-blockers and hydralazine. Sodium nitroprusside risks fetal toxicity and should not be used
- Consider delivering fetus (caesarian section).

ute MI in pregnancy

ute MI in pregnancy is rare, occurring in 1 per 10,000. Increasing
cidence may be due to rising maternal age. However, mortality is high
37–50%) particularly if the infarct occurs late in pregnancy.

Diagnosis is made using conventional criteria (📖 p.48). Troponin I is
not affected by normal pregnancy and is the marker of choice for myocardial necrosis in pregnancy.

☼ Acute management

There are few data to guide treatment. The risk from MI needs to be
weighed against the risks of treatment (to both mother and fetus).
- Aspirin 75 mg od
- Beta-blockers.

⚠ Systemic thrombolysis should not be given late in pregnancy because
of the risk of premature labour and potentially catastrophic bleeding.
However, in the presence of a large anterolateral acute MI, thrombolysis
should be considered if primary angioplasty is not available, since the
consequence of not treating carries such a high risk of maternal and fetal
demise.

- Primary PCI is probably the treatment of choice in a large AMI, since
  the consequence of not treating carry such a high risk of both maternal
  and fetal death. Although there are little data on the use of newer
  antiplatelet agents in pregnancy, there are reports of successful
  completion of pregnancy following primary angioplasty.

Pulmonary embolism in pregnancy

Venous thromboembolism is the second commonest cause of maternal
death, and poor management is implicated in many. Appropriate investigations should not be withheld because of pregnancy. Patients should be
anticoagulated pending confirmed diagnosis. CT scan and perfusion scans
carry a low risk to the fetus and should not be withheld.

☼ Acute management

- Low molecular weight heparin can be used but altered pharmacokinetics
  in pregnancy mean that doses may need to be altered according to levels
  of anti-Xa (0.6–1.0 units/mL)
- For life-threatening massive PE, consider (after specialist advice)
  intra-pulmonary thrombolysis, catheter (percutaneous) disruption of
  embolus, or surgical thrombectomy
- Where embolic episodes continue despite therapeutic anti-coagulation,
  consider a temporary caval filter.

Valvular heart disease in pregnancy

Mitral stenosis

Increased heart rate (decreased diastolic filling time) and increase circulating volume both serve to increase left atrial pressure and ma, precipitate acute pulmonary oedema. New or rapid AF will have similar effects.

Treatment
- Diuretics (avoid excessive diuresis—risk of hypovolaemia)
- Beta-blockers for rate control
- Anticoagulate with heparin (if AF and/or left atrial dilatation)
- Percutaneous (balloon) mitral valvuloplasty for severe mitral stenosis that is refractory to medical treatment.

Aortic stenosis

Usually due to a bicuspid aortic valve. The increased cardiac output required early in pregnancy can lead to problems due to the fixed LV outflow. Symptoms include SOB, syncope, chest pain. When these occur with severe aortic stenosis, consider delivery or palliative balloon valvuloplasty.

Valvular regurgitation

Mitral and aortic regurgitation are generally well tolerated during pregnancy, and the decreased afterload is often beneficial in reducing the degree of regurgitation. When symptoms occur, diuretics are the mainstay of treatment. ACE inhibitors should be avoided.

rhythmias in pregnancy

ormonal and haemodynamic changes may predispose pregnant women
to arrhythmias and may also render clinically silent paroxysmal tachycardias symptomatic. Note that DC cardioversion is safe in pregnancy.

Re-entry tachycardias

- Treat as for non-pregnant (📖 p.150)
- Vagal manoeuvres
- Adenosine, verapamil, flecainide have been used successfully
- DC cardioversion for severe haemodynamic compromise.

AF and atrial flutter

- Underlying cardiac disease likely and should be investigated
- Cardiovert if compromised and <24 hour duration
- Anticoagulate with low molecular weight heparin
- Beta-blockers to control rate
- Involve cardiologist and high risk obstetrician.

Ventricular tachycardia

- DC cardioversion acutely
- Requires further evaluation
- Subsequent management depends on underlying disease
- Involve cardiologist and high risk obstetrician.

Hypertension in pregnancy

Hypertension in pregnancy (BP >140 systolic or 90 mmHg diastolic) be considered in 3 categories:
- Chronic hypertension
- Gestational hypertension
- Pre-eclampsia.

Control of chronic hypertension i.e. diagnosed prior to or in early pregnancy may deteriorate and may require alteration to treatment. For example, ACE inhibitors are contraindicated in pregnancy and should be discontinued prior to conception. Gestational hypertension occurs late in pregnancy (last trimester). Pre-eclampsia tends to occur in younger women with onset after 20 weeks gestation. Abrupt onset oedema and proteinuria with raised plasma uric acid distinguish pre-eclampsia from chronic hypertension. Resolution following delivery is the rule.

Anti-hypertensive drugs used in pregnancy:

▶ Obtain expert advice.
- Methyldopa (250 mg TDS po initially) and/or hydralazine (5–10 mg IV, repeated after 30 minutes in severe hypertension) with calcium antagonists and beta-blockers as second line agents
- Magnesium sulphate in pre-eclampsia to prevent convulsions
- Avoid nitroprusside because of fetal toxicity.

Anticoagulation in pregnancy

Anticoagulation in pregnancy, particularly for prosthetic valves presents a difficult problem, with few data available for guidance. Warfarin risks teratogenicity (first trimester), fetal haemorrhage (especially in third trimester) and fetal loss throughout pregnancy. Heparin use has been implicated in prosthetic valve thrombosis. LMW heparin is preferred to unfractionated heparin, because anti-Xa levels can be monitored. It should be given as a BD regime.

The three main options are:
1. Heparin/LMW heparin plus aspirin throughout pregnancy.
2. Warfarin throughout pregnancy, changing to heparin at 38 weeks.
3. Heparin/LMW heparin plus aspirin in 1st trimester, changing to warfarin until 38 weeks when heparin is recommenced.

▶ Specialist advice should be sought and decisions made after consideration of case-specific issues.

cardioversion in pregnancy

- Place a wedge under the right hip to avoid IVC compression*
- Use lowest energy shock
- Direct the paddles away from fetus
- No reports of iatrogenic fetal VF
- …but, check fetal heart rate post-cardioversion.

* Procedures or investigations that usually require the patient to be supine should be done in a lateral position or with the aid of a wedge to support the pelvis and avoid IVC compression, by the gravid uterus, with consequent syncope.

Adult congenital heart disease

Introduction *218*
Atrial septal defect (ASD) *220*
Ventricular septal defect (VSD) *222*
Atrioventricular septal defect (AVSD)   *224*
Patent ductus arteriosus (PDA)   *224*
Aortic coarctation *226*
Transposition of the great arteries (TGA) *228*
Congenitally corrected transposition of the
    great arteries (ccTGA) *230*
Tetralogy of Fallot (ToF) *232*
The single ventricle *234*
The patient after Fontan operation *236*
The cyanosed patient *237*
Eisenmenger syndrome   *238*
Arrhythmias *239*
Syncope *240*
Heart failure *240*
Glossary of surgical procedures *242*

Introduction

Congenital heart disease occurs in about 0.8% of newborn infants. In UK, with a population of about 60 million, it is thought that there are least 150,000 adults with congenital heart disease. This number will gro in future as more children survive to adulthood and this has importan implications for physicians practicing in adult medicine.

Common presentations in emergency situations include:
• Arrhythmia
• Heart failure
• Endocarditis.

—all with high mortality. Special expertise is needed for optimal management.

Atrial septal defect (ASD)

An ASD is a direct communication between the atria that permits b‍‍‍
flow (usually from left to right atrium). There is subsequent enlargem‍‍‍
of the right atrium and ventricle and increased pulmonary blood flow.

The unoperated patient

Clinical features result from:
- Increased pulmonary blood flow
- Inability to increase cardiac output adequately because of the systemic to pulmonary shunting
- Paradoxical thromboembolism
- AF or flutter, related to right atrial dilatation.

Presentation
- Many are asymptomatic
- Symptomatic adults usually present with SOB or palpitation age 20–40
- ① May present as an emergency with stroke, heart failure or fast AF.

Signs
- Fixed splitting of the 2nd heart sound
- Pulmonary ejection murmur (due to increased flow)
- Cyanosis (uncommon; occurs in large defects with pulmonary hypertension).

Investigations
CXR: Cardiomegaly, right atrial dilatation & prominent pulmonary arteries are common with large shunts.
ECG: Right axis deviation and incomplete RBBB are typical findings in patients with significant defects.
Atrial arrhythmia (AF, flutter).

Management
- Acute management of stroke, heart failure or AF as in the non-ACHD setting
- An ASD that gives rise to right ventricular enlargement should be closed either surgically or with a percutaneous technique. This does not need to be done urgently
- If large defect, with established pulmonary hypertension, cyanosis ± Eisenmenger syndrome, closure may be too hazardous.

The operated patient

After ASD closure patients are usually symptom-free. However, they can present with atrial arrhythmias and heart failure especially when the defect has been closed late in life and the pulmonary artery pressure has been elevated prior to surgery. Complete heart block or sinus node dysfunction can also occur after closure.

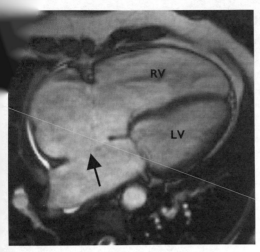

Cardiac magnetic resonance image of an atrial septal defect. Note the partial absence of atrial septum (arrowed) and the dilated RV.

Ventricular septal defect (VSD)

A VSD permits blood flow between the ventricles (usually from left to r
leading to an increase in pulmonary blood flow and enlargement of the
atrium and ventricle. The size of the VSD and the pulmonary vascular res
tance determine the degree and direction of the shunt.

The unoperated patient—problems
- Pulmonary hypertension if large defect (significant left-to-right shunt); may
  become permanent due to chronic pulmonary vascular changes
- Cyanosis occurs when ↑pulmonary vascular resistance eventually leads to
  a right-to-left shunt (Eisenmenger syndrome, 📖 p.238)
- Heart failure from left ventricular dysfunction due to long-term volume
  overload
- Atrial and ventricular arrhythmias due to chamber enlargement
- Aortic regurgitation (📖 p.114), even with small VSDs, due to the
  potential proximity of the defect to the aortic valve
- Increased risk of endocarditis (📖 p.96)—all patients with VSDs
- Pregnancy is usually well tolerated in patients with a small or moderate
  VSD but carries a high risk in patients with pulmonary vascular disease
  (Eisenmenger syndrome, 📖 p.238).

ⓘ *Acute presentation*
Endocarditis, atrial and ventricular arrhythmias or heart failure.

Signs
- Coarse pansystolic heart murmur at left sternal border ('the louder the
  VSD murmur, the smaller the defect')
- Left ± right ventricular heave
- Cyanosis if Eisenmenger syndrome has developed (📖 p.238).

Investigations
CXR: Normal (small defect), cardiomegaly, ↑pulmonary marking (moderate
defect), oligemic lung fields, enlarged proximal pulmonary arteries (large
defect with Eisenmenger syndrome).
ECG: Broad P wave, signs of LV enlargement or RV hypertrophy
(Eisenmenger syndrome), arrhythmia.

Management
- Acute presenting problems managed as in the non-ACHD setting
- Nearly all VSDs should be closed to alleviate LV enlargement, prevent the
  development of irreversible pulmonary artery disease and to reduce the
  risk of aortic regurgitation and bacterial endocarditis (exception: small
  uncomplicated VSDs).

The operated patient
- Usually symptom-free but can present with atrial or ventricular arrhythmia
  or heart failure, especially when the defect has been closed late in life and
  the pulmonary artery pressure has been elevated
- Complete heart block can occur after closure
- Pulmonary vascular disease can progress, regress or remain stable
  post-operatively.

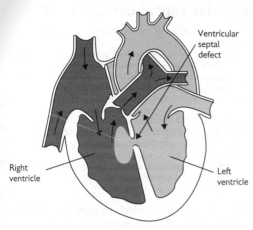

Ventricular
septal
defect

Right
ventricle

Left
ventricle

Diagram of a ventricular septal defect.

Restrictive and non-restrictive VSD

Restrictive VSDs 'restrict' the flow across the defect. They are thus small VSDs (<$\frac{1}{3}$ of the aortic root diameter), and there is a pressure gradient between the left and right ventricles. RV pressures and pulmonary resistance are normal.

Moderately restrictive VSDs are about ½ the size of the aortic valve, with moderate–severe shunting early in the disease process. RV pressures are increased, but not to systemic levels. Pulmonary resistance can be raised, and the left atrium and ventricle can be dilated due to volume overload.

Non-restrictive VSDs are large, resulting in equal left and right ventricular pressures. The pulmonary circulation is subject to systemic pressures and significantly increased flow, which leads to increased pulmonary resistance within the first years of life. This reduces the left-to-right shunt and continued pulmonary vascular changes ultimately result in reversal of the shunt (right-to-left) and Eisenmenger syndrome (🔲 p.238).

Atrioventricular septal defect (AVSD)

The term AVSD covers a spectrum of anomalies at the junction between the atria and ventricles:
- The defect can consist only of an ASD (ostium primum) or can include an inlet-type VSD, which can be restrictive or non-restrictive
- Additionally, the atrioventricular valves (mitral and tricuspid) are often abnormal and can be regurgitant
- AVSDs occur in 35% of patients with Down syndrome.

Physiological consequences
- Generally similar to the condition of an isolated ASD or VSD and relate to the degree of left-to-right shunting and the presence or absence of pulmonary hypertension
- The abnormality of the AV valves can result in additional problems, including heart failure and atrial arrhythmia.

Repair
Following AVSD repair, mitral or tricuspid regurgitation or stenosis, subaortic stenosis and complete AV block can occur.

Patent ductus arteriosus (PDA)

A PDA represents a persistent communication between the descending aorta and the proximal left pulmonary artery.
- There is a left-to-right shunt with increased pulmonary flow leading to enlargement of the left atrium and ventricle
- Small ducts cause a murmur without haemodynamic effects
- Large ducts lead to pulmonary hypertension and pulmonary vascular disease, ultimately resulting in Eisenmenger syndrome and a right-to-left shunt across the PDA into the *descending* aorta. This results in differential cyanosis (reduced lower body oxygen saturations with maintained upper body saturation).

Signs
Continuous (systolic and diastolic) murmur at upper left sternal border; long ejection systolic murmur with small PDAs.

Acute presentation
① Rare—endarteritis (like endocarditis) is the main cause.

Management
- Endarteritis managed as for endocarditis in the non-ACHD setting (📖 p.96)
- Closure of PDA is indicated if left heart enlarged or when a murmur is present (to reduce the small risk of endarteritis).

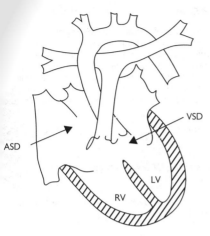

Diagram of an atrioventricular septal defect.

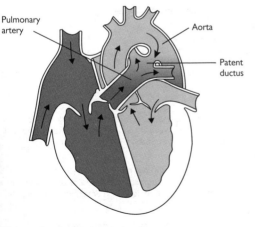

Diagram of a patent ductus arteriosus.

Aortic coarctation

Aortic coarctation is a narrowing of the aorta in the region of t~
mentum arteriosum, just distal to the left subclavian artery. If sever~
lower body relies on collateral vessels via the intercostal arteries
perfusion. Complete occlusion is also possible. A 'simple' coarctation~
one without other cardiac lesions. A 'complex' coarctation is associate~
with other defects such as a VSD or left sided obstructive lesion (e.g
aortic stenosis). At least 50% of patients with coarctation have a bicuspid
aortic valve.

The unoperated patient

Risks
- Upper body hypertension
- Heart failure from long-standing LV pressure load
- Aortic rupture or dissection
- Infective endocarditis
- Stroke from an associated ruptured berry aneurysm + hypertension
- Premature coronary artery disease.

Signs
- Upper limb hypertension and differential arm–leg pulses. Blood
  pressure measurement in the right arm and a leg is necessary in all new
  patients with hypertension). A pressure difference of ≥20 mmHg may
  suggest coarctation
- Continuous murmur in the interscapular region.

Investigations
ECG: Left ventricular hypertrophy.
CXR: 'Three sign' caused by narrowing of the aorta at the site of coarctation
with dilatation of the vessel before and after the coarctation, 'rib notching'
caused by erosions of the inferior edge of the ribs by enlarged intercostal
arteries.
CT: Good visualization of location and severity using contrast and recon-
structed images.
MRI: Excellent visualization of anatomy, possible aneurysm formation and,
using contrast angiography, 3D visualization of the geometry and col-
laterals. Velocity measurements can assess the degree of stenosis.

Management
- Acute consequences managed as in the non-ACHD setting
- Surgical repair or stenting of the stenosis may be indicated if significant
  gradient across coarctation (>20 mmHg) ± proximal hypertension.

The operated patient
- ✪: Re-coarctation and aneurysm formation (often intercostal) at the
  site of repair are not uncommon; aneurysm rupture presents acutely!
- Other aortic wall complications are frequent
- Hypertension can persist or develop in adulthood and needs to be
  treated aggressively because of the risk of atherosclerosis
- The need for endocarditis prophylaxis remains.

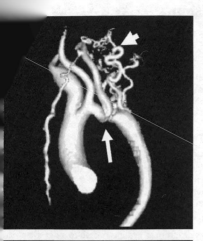

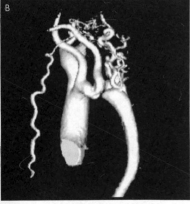

Magnetic resonance angiogram of aortic coarctation.
(A) AP view showing site of coarctation (long arrow), enlarged head and neck
vessels and extensive collateral circulation to the descending aorta (short arrow).
(B) rotated view showing complete nature of coarctation.

Transposition of the great arteries

- The aorta arises from the RV and the pulmonary artery from the L
- Can be associated with other lesions, e.g. VSD or coarctation
- Incompatible with life without treatment in the first few days.

Atrial switch operation

- The most common operation amongst adults with TGA is an 'atrial switch operation' (either Mustard or Senning operation, 📖 p.244, 245)
- The atrial blood flow has been 'switched' in a way that the RV receives the pulmonary venous blood and the LV receives the systemic venous blood, however, the RV remains the systemic ventricle.

Arterial switch operation (📖 p.242)

The 'atrial switch operation' has been replaced by the 'arterial switch operation' in which the aorta and pulmonary artery are switched to the anatomically correct position, with the LV connected to the aorta and the RV to the pulmonary artery (the LV becomes the systemic ventricle).

The patient after 'atrial switch operation'

- There is a significant morbidity from arrhythmia related to extensive atrial surgery: bradyarrhythmias (sinus node dysfunction, slow junctional escape rhythm) and tachyarrhythmias (atrial flutter) occur
- RV dysfunction is common, as it is not built to support the systemic circulation
- Tricuspid regurgitation can accompany right heart failure
- Obstruction of the atrial pathways ('baffle obstruction') can lead to systemic or pulmonary venous congestion.

Signs

- Systolic heart murmur from tricuspid regurgitation
- Heart failure
- Peripheral oedema and ascites from systemic venous congestion.

Investigations

- *ECG*—Right axis deviation, RV hypertrophy, atrial arrhythmias
- *CXR*—Cardiomegaly, pulmonary congestion.

Management

- The complexity of arrhythmia management, including pacing, and the difficulty in assessing RV function requires a specialist centre
- Thorough assessment of RV and tricuspid valve function, heart rhythm and the function of the intra-atrial venous pathways is paramount
- Therapeutic options include catheterization techniques (balloon dilatation and stenting for pathway obstructions), surgical procedures (tricuspid valve repair/replacement or even conversion to the arterial switch operation, for selected patients)
- The end of the therapeutic spectrum is heart transplantation.

❶ If pacing is required for bradycardia, this must be performed by experts, as placement of the leads within the atria and into the left (pulmonary) ventricle can be immensely difficult.

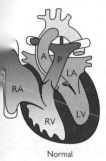

Normal

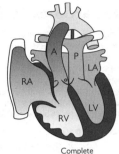

Complete
transposition

The patient after 'arterial switch operation'

- Arrhythmias are less common and ventricular function is usually well preserved
- Suture lines in the pulmonary trunk can cause stenosis
- Peripheral pulmonary artery stenosis can be caused by the position of the pulmonary bifurcation anterior to the ascending aorta
- Progressive dilatation of the aortic root (former pulmonary root) can cause aortic regurgitation
- Coronary artery reimplantation may result in ostial coronary stenosis and ischaemia.

Signs

- Ejection systolic heart murmur from pulmonary artery stenosis
- Diastolic heart murmur from aortic regurgitation.

Investigations

- *ECG*—Signs of myocardial ischaemia and RV hypertrophy.

Management

The main issue in the care of patients after arterial switch operation is to exclude significant pulmonary artery stenosis, myocardial ischaemia, and aortic valve regurgitation. All these situations may warrant intervention.

Congenitally corrected transposition
the great arteries (ccTGA)

In ccTGA the ventricles are 'inverted'. Systemic venous return enters
left ventricle which than ejects into the pulmonary artery. Pulmona
venous return enters the right ventricle which fills the aorta. The circula
tion is therefore 'physiologically corrected' but the right ventricle is
supporting the systemic circulation.

ccTGA is often associated with other defects e.g. systemic (tricuspid)
atrioventricular valve abnormalities and regurgitation, VSD, subpulmonary
stenosis and complete heart block. ccTGA can occur with dextrocardia.

The unoperated patient

- Progressive RV dysfunction is common as it is not designed to support
  the systemic circulation
- Risk of bradyarrhythmias (complete AV block) and tachyarrhythmias
  (atrial arrhythmia 📖 p.140–148 or SVT secondary to WPW syndrome,
  📖 p.152)
- Patients with a VSD and pulmonary stenosis can be cyanotic.

The operated patient

Patients may have been operated for their associated lesions. Common
procedures are:
- VSD closure
- Implantation of a conduit from the LV to the pulmonary artery
- Systemic (tricuspid) atrioventricular valve replacement.

A 'corrective procedure' would be the 'double switch operation' (combination of an atrial and arterial switch operation). As for atrial switch
operations, atrial arrhythmias are common following this.

Signs

Systolic heart murmur—VSD, pulmonary stenosis or tricuspid regurgitation may be difficult to differentiate.

Investigations

- ECG—Arrhythmia (complete AV block, atrial arrhythmia)
- CXR—Dextrocardia (20% of patients), cardiomegaly.

Management

- Preservation of systemic (right) ventricular function is crucial
- Tricuspid regurgitation has to be treated surgically (valve replacement)
  before ventricular dysfunction becomes irreversible
- Symptomatic bradycardia or chronotropic incompetence is an
  indication for pacemaker implantation
- Atrial arrhythmias are common after atrial surgery or with severe
  tricuspid regurgitation. They are not well tolerated in the setting of a
  systemic RV, especially with dysfunction and tricuspid regurgitation
- Endocarditis prophylaxis is necessary in all patients.

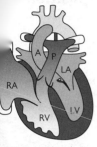

Normal

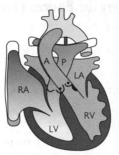

Congenitally corrected
transposition

Tetralogy of Fallot (ToF)

ToF consists of:
• A large VSD
• Right ventricular outflow tract obstruction (RVOTO)
• Right ventricular hypertrophy
• An overriding aorta.

The physiological consequences are determined by the degree of RVOTO which in turn determines the magnitude of pulmonary blood flow. Significant RVOTO leads to a right-to-left shunt and cyanosis. Survival to adulthood in unoperated patients with ToF is rare.

The operated or repaired patient

• Surgical repair includes VSD closure and relief of the RVOTO and may involve patching of the pulmonary valve annulus, which can lead to pulmonary regurgitation
• Pulmonary regurgitation in turn may lead to right ventricular enlargement and dysfunction and is associated with VT and sudden death. However, the majority of patients tolerate the regurgitation well
• Atrial arrhythmias are not uncommon especially if right atrial enlargement is present.

Signs

Diastolic murmur (pulmonary or aortic regurgitation), systolic murmur (residual RVOTO or VSD).

Investigations

• *ECG*—complete RBBB, QRS prolongation
• *CXR*—cardiomegaly.

Management

• ⑦ Pulmonary valve replacement should be considered for patients with severe pulmonary regurgitation and right ventricular dilatation. New percutaneous techniques, using stent-mounted pericardial valves, show promise in selected patients.
• ① The development of arrhythmias (VT and atrial flutter/fibrillation) warrants both full electrophysiologic assessment and thorough review of the haemodynamics.

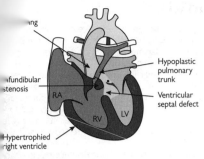

...ing

...fundibular stenosis

RA

RV   LV

Hypertrophied right ventricle

Hypoplastic pulmonary trunk

Ventricular septal defect

Diagram showing a heart with Tetralogy of Fallot.

The single ventricle

Hearts with an 'anatomically' or 'functionally' single ventricle receive systemic and pulmonary venous blood in 'one' ventricle, which can be predominantly left or right ventricular morphology. The ventricle pumps blood into the pulmonary artery (when not atretic) and the aorta.

The best situation is when blood flows unrestricted into a well functioning ventricle, which pumps an equivalent amount of blood into the lungs and systemic circulation. In this situation, excessive pulmonary blood flow is avoided by an obstruction of the pulmonary outflow tract. If pulmonary outflow tract obstruction is not present, excessive blood flow into the lungs will lead to pulmonary hypertension and the Eisenmenger syndrome (📖 p. 238).

Severe pulmonary outflow tract obstruction with reduced pulmonary blood flow causes cyanosis (📖 p. 237).

Surgery in patients with single ventricles is always palliative and aims to secure adequate pulmonary and systemic blood flow and maintain systemic ventricular function.

Surgery for single ventricles

- Aorto-pulmonary shunts (📖 p. 242) are commonly performed in early infancy to improve pulmonary blood flow. As the single ventricle continues to pump blood into both the aorta and pulmonary arteries, volume overload remains a problem
- Pulmonary artery banding is performed when pulmonary blood flow is unobstructed, to protect against pulmonary hypertension
- Systemic venous to pulmonary artery connections like the Glenn shunt (📖 p. 244) or the Fontan operation (📖 p. 242) are performed as definitive palliations to improve pulmonary blood flow and separate the pulmonary from the systemic circulation while unloading the systemic ventricle.

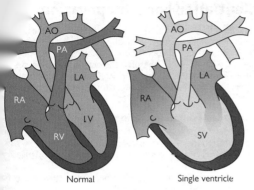

Normal

Single ventricle

Diagram showing a normal (two-ventricle) heart and a heart with a single ventricle.

The patient after Fontan operation

Many adult patients with a single ventricle have undergone Fontan o͟
tions (📖 p. 242). Following this operation, all systemic venous retu͟
diverted to the pulmonary circulation without employing a subpulmo͟
ventricle. Blood flow to the lungs, therefore, is only driven by syste͟
venous pressure. 'Fontan patients' are at risk of various complicatio͟
related to surgery and/or the abnormal circulatory physiology persistin͟
after surgery.

Complications after Fontan operation

Arrhythmias
- Sinus node dysfunction may warrant pacemaker implantation
- Atrial flutter/fibrillation related to scarring from surgery, or to atrial
  distension from high venous pressure.

:⚙: Atrial arrhythmias in 'Fontan patients' need prompt treatment as they
can cause profound haemodynamic deterioration.

Thromboembolism
Associated with sluggish venous blood flow.

Protein losing enteropathy (PLE)
Occurs in 10% of 'Fontan patients' and is characterized by intestina͟
protein loss leading to low serum protein levels and subsequently to
peripheral oedema and ascites.

Deterioration of ventricular function
This is the 'natural' history, especially if the ventricle is of RV morphology.

Hepatic dysfunction
Resulting from high hepatic venous pressure.

Cyanosis
From persistent right-to-left shunting.

Signs
- A 'good' 'Fontan patient' has no murmurs and a single 2nd heart sound
  (systolic murmurs can indicate atrioventricular valve incompetence)
- Peripheral oedema (heart failure or PLE).

Investigations
- *ECG*—arrhythmia
- *CXR*—cardiomegaly, atrial enlargement
- *Bloods*—abnormal LFT, low protein/albumin suggestive of PLE.

Management
- 'Fontan patients' are one of the most challenging group of patients in
  cardiology and require close follow up by tertiary centre specialists
- Treatment aims to maintain optimal pulmonary and systemic
  circulation and to preserve ventricular function.

...yanosed patient

...is is common in ACHD 2° to right-to-left shunting or decreased ...nary blood flow. The resulting hypoxaemia leads to adaptive ...anisms to increase oxygen delivery to the tissues. These include a ...tward shift in the oxy-haemoglobin binding curve and ↑haemoglobin ...ncentration (secondary erythrocytosis, not polycythaemia).

Symptoms related to hypoxia include SOB at rest or on exertion and chest pain. Other symptoms result from the multi-organ consequences.

The multi-organ consequences of cyanosis

Haematological
- Erythrocytosis
- Iron deficiency (high demand, dietary or induced by inappropriate venesections)
- Coagulopathy, bleeding diathesis, thrombocytopenia, impaired clotting function.

Neurological
- Brain injury from paradoxical embolism, haemorrhage, abscesses.

Renal
- Hypoxaemia induced glomerulopathy (haematuria, proteinuria)
- Nephrolithiasis (uric acid).

Rheumatological
- Gout
- Osteoarthropathy.

Management

Venesection in cyanosed patients—only if:
- Severe symptoms of 'hyperviscosity syndrome' (e.g. headache, dizziness, fatigue, visual disturbances, tinnitus and myalgia) are present after 'correcting' dehydration and haematocrit >65%
- Surgery is planned and haematocrit >65%.

Venesection procedure
- 250–500 mL of blood to be removed over 45 min
- Volume replacement with 5% **dextrose**
- Use IV 'air filters' (to reduce the risk of systemic air embolus)
- Blood pressure and heart rate monitoring are required.

Iron deficiency
Needs oral or IV iron supplements.

Anticoagulation
No general consensus on routine anticoagulation—requires specialist consideration.

Eisenmenger syndrome

Eisenmenger syndrome is a pathophysiological condition resulting ACHD. Uncorrected left-to-right shunting and progressive pulmo hypertension eventually leads to reversal of the shunt and cyanosis w right sided pressure exceeds systemic. VSD, AVSD and large PDAs responsible for 80% of cases. Eisenmenger patients exhibit signs ar symptoms related to chronic cyanosis (📖 p. 242) and are at risk o complications related to pulmonary hypertension (📖 p. 196).

Signs
Cyanosis, loud 2nd heart sound, no murmur from original lesion.

Investigations
- *ECG*—right ventricular hypertrophy
- *CXR*—oligaemic lung fields, enlarged proximal pulmonary arteries.

Acute presentation
- Progressive heart failure
- Atrial arrhythmias
- Angina
- Syncope and sudden cardiac death
- Haemoptysis and intrapulmonary bleeding
- Pulmonary artery thrombosis (embolism or *in situ* thrombosis).

Management
Haemoptysis/intrapulmonary bleeding
- Bed rest
- CXR and CT scan to determine extent of haemorrhage
- FBC (repeatedly if continuous bleeding is suspected)
- Monitoring of oxygen saturation, blood pressure, diuresis
- Embolization of culprit vessels identified by angiography.

Anticoagulation
- To prevent recurrent embolic events
- No general consensus on routine anticoagulation (bleeding diathesis).

Treatment of pulmonary hypertension
While pulmonary vasodilator therapy with agents such as prostacyclin analogues and endothelin antagonists are established forms of therapy in *primary* pulmonary hypertension, placebo controlled trials on the efficacy and safety of these drugs in Eisenmenger patients are under way. Early observational studies are encouraging.

Rules in the care of Eisenmenger patients
- Avoid *hypovolaemia* and *dehydration*
- Avoid *non cardiac surgery* and general *anaesthesia* if possible
- General anaesthesia always needs to be performed by an experienced anaesthetist
- Post-operative care in ICU
- Use IV 'air filters' or 'bubble trap' for any intravenous line.

rrhythmias

ythmias are very common in adults with ACHD as part of the ural' history or resulting from surgery and/or progressive residual emodynamic lesions. Arrhythmias in these patients are associated with gnificant morbidity and mortality. Both detection and treatment of rrhythmia in adults with ACHD can be challenging.

⊃: Atypical atrial flutter and intra-atrial re-entry tachycardia (IART)

IART is usually caused by atrial stretch or previous extensive atrial sur- gery (Fontan, Mustard, Senning). Intra-atrial excitation circuits around electrical barriers such as scars and suture lines cause rapid atrial heart rate or flutter. Atrioventricular conduction may be normal in relatively young adults, allowing for a fast 1:1 conduction and a fast ventricular rate leading to haemodynamic compromise.

Treatment

Radiofrequency ablation can block the circuits and potentially treat the arrhythmia. Electrophysiologists with special expertise in CHD are required for these demanding procedures.

Ventricular tachycardia (VT)

VT is commonly associated with previous ventricular surgery or long- standing abnormal ventricular load:
- Previous VSD closure
- ToF repair (prolonged QRS duration is a risk marker)
- Pulmonary regurgitation and right ventricular enlargement
- Single ventricles
- Mustard or Senning repairs
- ccTGA.

Indications for ICD implantation in congenital heart disease are awaited.

General considerations for the treatment of arrhythmias

- Obtain as much information on the patient as possible
- Assess the patient thoroughly for signs of heart failure and infection
- Obtain a 12-lead ECG & compare with previous ECGs (ACHD patients often have a broad QRS complex)
- Only transfer patients to a tertiary centre once stable
- Seek expert advice early.

Syncope

Syncope is always a matter of concern in patients with ACHD espe
if they are cyanosed or have pulmonary hypertension.

Causes for syncope in ACHD
- Tachyarrhythmia
- Bradycardia from sinus node dysfunction, AV block
- Pulmonary embolism
- Severe pulmonary hypertension
- Severe obstructive lesion (valve stenosis etc.)
- Aortic dissection, rupture
- Myocardial ischaemia
- Hypotension (drug induced?)
- Vasovagal.

▶ Any syncope in a patient with congenital heart disease should initiate
thorough electrophysiological and haemodynamic assessment and ideally
should involve an expert in ACHD!

⊙ Heart failure

In any patient with ACHD disease presenting with heart failure, an acute
underlying cause has to be excluded. Common ones are:
- Arrhythmia
- Infection
- Ischaemia.

Adult patients with ACHD often have very finely balanced haemodynamics with minimal cardiac reserve and even minor changes in their condition can cause severe deterioration.

Lesions that present with left or 'systemic' heart failure
- Left sided valve disease (mitral and aortic valve)
- TGA after Mustard or Senning repair and ccTGA
- Systemic left ventricular dysfunction in older ToF patients.

Lesions that present with right or 'subpulmonary' heart failure
- Fontan patients
- Pulmonary hypertension/Eisenmenger syndrome
- Right sided valve disease (tricuspid and pulmonary valve)
- Mustard with obstruction of intra-atrial pathways
- Elderly patients with late repair or unrepaired ASD.

Medical treatment
▶ Seek expert advice early.

- Find the cause
- Restore sinus rhythm as soon as possible in compromised patients
- Medical treatment will not affect anatomic lesions
- Standard treatment for heart failure, including diuretics, but be
  cautious with vasodilator therapy.

Heart failure treatment—considerations for ACHD patients

	Pros	Cons
Loop diuretics	• Effective, improves symptoms	• Rapidly reduces preload • Caution in Fontan patients
Spironolactone	• Effective, improves symptoms	

ACE inhibitors	• Effective to reduce hypertension.
	• Unknown long term benefits on heart function
		• Little evidence to improve heart function.
		• Caution if
		  • Preload dependant
		  • Obstructive lesion present
		  • Renal dysfunction
		  • Pulmonary hypertension

Beta-blocker	• Anti-arrhythmic • Good for heart rate control	• Caution in bradycardia.
Digoxin	• Rate control in atrial flutter	

Modified from *Adult Congenital Heart Disease: A Practical Guide.* Gatzoulis et al. (eds). BMJ Books, Blackwell Publishing Group (with permission).

⑦ Glossary of surgical procedures

Arterial switch operation or Jatene procedure

Operation for TGA patients, switch of the great arteries to bring th
aorta in the former pulmonary artery position and the pulmonary artery
in the former aortic position. The coronary arteries have to be trans-
posed from the aortic root to the former pulmonary artery root (neo
aorta). Ultimately, the left ventricle will perfuse the aorta and the right
ventricle will perfuse the pulmonary artery.

Bentall operation

Replacement of the ascending aorta and aortic valve with a composite
graft (conduit) and valve and re-implantation of the coronary arteries
into the conduit.

Brock procedure

Palliative procedure for ToF patients. Closed resection of right ventricular musculature from the outflow tract using a biopsy like instrument and
dilatation (valvotomy) of the pulmonary valve.

Classic Blalock–Taussig (BT) shunt

Subclavian artery to ipsilateral pulmonary artery anastomosis (direct end-
to-side junction).

Modified Blalock–Taussig (BT) shunt

Same shunt using a prosthetic graft.

Damus–Kaye–Stansel operation

Operation connecting aorta and pulmonary artery in a side-to-side
fashion to provide unrestricted blood flow from the systemic ventricle to
the aorta. For patients with single ventricles and transposition of the
great arteries and restrictive VSD leading to subaortic stenosis.

Fontan operation

Palliative operation for patients with 'single' ventricle physiology
(📖 p.234). Diversion of the systemic venous return to the lung without
interposition of a subpulmonary ventricle. Leads to volume unloading of
the 'single' ventricle and ideally to normalization of the arterial oxygen
saturation.

Multiple variations of the procedure exists regarding the type of
connection between the systemic veins and the pulmonary arteries:

- **Classic Fontan:** Connection between right atrium and pulmonary
  artery
- **Extracardiac Fontan:** Inferior vena cava connected to pulmonary
  artery via an extracardiac conduit combined with a Glenn shunt
  (opposite)
- **Bjoerk or RA–RV Fontan:** Valved conduit between the right atrium
  and the right ventricle
- **Total cavopulmonary connection (TCPC):** Inferior vena cava
  connected to pulmonary artery via an intra atrial tunnel (also called
  lateral tunnel), combined with a Glenn shunt to the SVC.

Total cavopulmonary connection (TCPC, lateral tunnel)

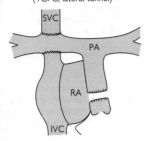

TCPC (Extracardiac conduit*)

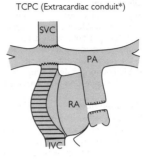

Atriopulmonary Fontan

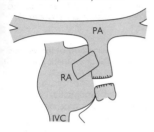

Classical Glenn

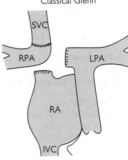

Bidirectional Glenn

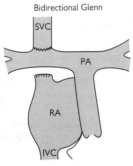

Bilateral bidirectional Glenn

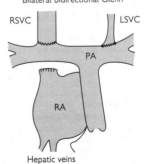

Glenn shunt

Superior vena cava (SVC) to pulmonary artery anastomosis.
- **Classical Glenn shunt:** Anastomosis of the superior vena cava to the distal right pulmonary artery with ligation of the SVC below the anastomosis and division of the proximal right pulmonary artery from the pulmonary bifurcation
- **Bidirectional Glenn shunt:** Anastomosis of the superior vena cava to the undivided pulmonary artery.

Konno operation

Complex repair and reconstruction of the left ventricular outflow tract for patients with tunnel-like subvalvar left ventricular outflow tract obstruction. The operation involves enlargement of the outflow tract by inserting a patch in the interventricular septum and aortic valve replacement as well as enlargement of the aortic annulus and the ascending aorta.

Lecompte manoeuvre

Manoeuvre that brings the pulmonary artery in a position anterior to the ascending aorta (part of the arterial switch operation or Jatene procedure).

Mustard operation

Atrial switch operation for patients with TGA: redirection of the venous blood to the contralateral ventricle using pericardial or synthetic patches.

Norwood operation

Initial palliative procedure for the treatment of hypoplastic left heart syndrome with aortic atresia and hypoplasia of the ascending aorta. Operation involves the reconstruction of 'neo-ascending' aorta using the pulmonary valve and trunk and the creation of an aorto-pulmonary shunt (usually modified BT shunt).

Pott's anastomosis shunt

Descending aorta to left pulmonary artery anastomosis.

Rastelli operation

Operation for patients with TGA, VSD and pulmonary stenosis, closure of the VSD in a way that the patch forms the left ventricular outflow tract to the aorta. The right ventricle is connected to the main pulmonary artery using a valved conduit.

Ross operation

Aortic valve replacement by transplantation of the patient's pulmonary valve into aortic position (pulmonary autograft) and by replacing the pulmonary valve using a homograft valve.
Major advantages:
- Potential of the 'neo-aortic' valve (former pulmonary valve) to grow in children
- No need for anticoagulation.

...ing operation

...al switch operation for patients with TGA, redirection of the venous
...od to the contralateral ventricle using the atrial wall and the septum.

...aterston shunt

Ascending aorta to right pulmonary artery anastomosis.

Acknowledgement

Figures on pages 229, 231, 233, and 243 are modified from *Adult congenital heart disease: a practical guide*. Gatzoulis et al. (eds). BMJ books, Blackwell Publishing Group (with permission).

Peri-operative care

Peri-operative issues 248
Pre-operative assessment 248
Predictors of risk 250
Determining risk 252
Need for coronary revascularization 252
Peri-operative issues in relation to
    specific conditions 254
Cardiac surgery 258

ⓘ Peri-operative issues

Cardiovascular complications of anaesthesia and surgery are common patients suffering from ischaemic heart disease, left ventricular dysfunction, arterial hypertension, and valvular heart disease.

Size of the problem

The National Confidential Enquiry into Peri-operative Death (NCEPOD) reveals that approximately 20,000 deaths within 30 days of surgery occur annually in England and Wales. Sixty percent of these patients have evidence of coronary heart disease and approximately 8,000 deaths have a cardiovascular cause.

In addition, estimates suggest 90,000 to 180,000 major peri-operative cardiovascular complications (MI, acute left ventricular failure, unstable angina, life-threatening arrhythmias). The high number of cardiovascular complications reflects the nature of surgery: a stress test that cannot easily be stopped once the operation has started.

Pre-operative risk assessment is therefore an important element of informed consent and also influences the strategy for anaesthesia and post-operative care. Collaboration between surgeons, anaesthetists and physicians, especially cardiologists, is essential to ensure optimal management.

Pre-operative assessment

Medical opinion is sought on diagnosis, clinical status and the appropriateness of the patient's current treatment. The medical opinion may conclude that further evaluation is required and/or recommend specific treatments e.g. revascularization or pacing prior to surgery.

Guided by this medical opinion, the anaesthetist can determine the patient's fitness for anaesthesia and surgery and develop a strategy for anaesthesia and post-operative care. This includes the extent of cardiovascular monitoring and the best location for post-operative care e.g. Intensive Care or High Dependency Unit. *Informed consent* will require consideration of the risks as well as the benefits of the procedure.

Predictors of risk

The risk of peri-operative cardiac complications relates to both the clinical status of the patient and the nature of the proposed surgery. The following stratification of predictors is based on the American College of Cardiology/American Heart Association guidelines. Clearly, the highest risk occurs when a patient with a 'major' clinical risk factor(s) undergoes a 'major' risk surgical procedure.

Predictors related to the patient

Major

- Unstable coronary syndromes
- Acute or recent MI
- Unstable or severe angina (Canadian class III or IV 🕮 p.255)
- Decompensated heart failure
- Significant arrhythmias
- High grade atrioventricular block
- Symptomatic ventricular arrhythmias
- Supraventricular arrhythmias with uncontrolled ventricular rate
- Severe valvular disease.

Intermediate

- Mild angina (Canadian Class I or II 🕮 p.255)
- Previous MI (history, pathological Q waves)
- Compensated or prior heart failure
- Diabetes mellitus
- Renal insufficiency.

Minor

- Advanced age
- Abnormal ECG (left ventricular hypertrophy, LBBB, ST-T segment abnormalities)
- Rhythm other than sinus
- Low functional capacity (inability to climb one flight of stairs)
- History of stroke
- Uncontrolled systemic hypertension.

Special considerations

- Severe hypertension with target organ involvement, left ventricular hypertrophy and strain
- Co-morbidity (not mentioned above)
- Obstructive airway disease
- Possible interactions between medication and anaesthetic agents
- Most cardiovascular drugs can be safely administered throughout the peri-operative period
- Angiotensin converting enzyme inhibitors and angiotensin receptor antagonists may have to be omitted on the morning of surgery to reduce the risk of intractable hypotension.

...dictors related to surgery

...jor (reported cardiac risk >5%)

Emergency major operation (particularly in the elderly)
Aortic and other major vascular surgery
- Peripheral vascular surgery
- Anticipated prolonged procedures with large fluid shifts and/or blood loss.

Intermediate (reported cardiac risk generally <5%)

- Carotid endarterectomy
- Head and neck surgery
- Intraperitoneal and intrathoracic surgery
- Orthopaedic surgery
- Prostate surgery.

Low risk

- Endoscopic procedures
- Superficial procedures
- Cataract surgery
- Breast surgery.

In addition, special consideration should be given to the following:

- Cardiovascular effect of aortic cross-clamping and de-clamping
- Gut handling leading to the release of inflammatory mediators
- Surgery likely to impair post-operative respiratory function.

Predictors related to the type of anaesthetic

There is a perception that in cardiac patients, spinal or epidural anaesthesia are safer than general anaesthesia. There is however no scientific evidence of reduced cardiac risk with these types of anaesthesia. Where spinal or epidural anaesthesia offer major advantages, monitoring needs to be extensive because of the possibility of rapid changes in vascular resistance due to autonomic blockade resulting in severe hypotension.

Local anaesthesia and regional anaesthesia (regional nerve blocks) are associated with a relatively low risk of post-operative cardiac events.

Determining risk

- Cardiac disease is not always clinically obvious, particularly where function is limited e.g. by arthritis or peripheral vascular disease
- Where potentially life-saving emergency surgery is required (e.g. ruptured aortic aneurysm, major trauma) it may be sufficient to identify risk and to anticipate and treat cardiac complications, with a view to further cardiac evaluation post-operatively
- In the non-emergency setting, patients with 'Major' clinical risk factors usually require further investigation and/or treatment
- Broadly speaking, patients with no more than 'Intermediate' clinical risk factors, a functional capacity that would allow them to walk up a hill or play a round of golf, and who are undergoing surgery of 'Intermediate' risk or less can proceed with a low probability of cardiac events
- Where functional capacity is low and/or a 'Major' risk procedure is to be undertaken, it is reasonable to proceed to non-invasive functional investigation (e.g. exercise ECG, pharmacologic stress echo-cardiography, stress radio nuclide ventriculography, or stress perfusion scintigraphy). Low reserve increases substantially the risk of cardiac complications after major surgery and further evaluation e.g. with coronary angiography may be indicated.

ⓘ Need for coronary revascularization

Coronary artery bypass surgery or percutaneous coronary intervention may be necessary in selected patients to decrease the risk of cardiac complications from anaesthesia and surgery. Current guidelines recommend that coronary revascularization, if indicated by conventional criteria (irrespective of planned non-cardiac surgery), should normally precede non-cardiac surgery. If coronary revascularization is not warranted for conventional clinical indications, revascularization should only be considered before high risk surgery (particularly major vascular surgery).

ⓘ Peri-operative issues in relation to specific conditions

Please read in conjunction with the patient-focussed approach (above).

Coronary artery disease

Coronary disease is the most frequent cause of cardiac complications from anaesthesia and surgery. In susceptible individuals, coronary events may be precipitated by haemodynamic perturbations (tachycardia, hypotension, hypertension), peri-operative hypoxaemia (especially nocturnal hypoxaemia after abdominal surgery), altered coagulation and post-operative anaemia.

Angina
- Well controlled angina increases the risk of anaesthesia and surgery but this increase is generally acceptable
- Unstable angina is an absolute contraindication to elective surgery and must be investigated pre-operatively as morbidity and mortality are unacceptably high.

Prior myocardial infarction
- The time that has elapsed between MI and proposed elective surgery is important. An interval of 3–6 months is generally advocated. Recently a delay of only 6 weeks has been regarded as acceptable in uncomplicated MI with no ischaemia on a stress test.
- Myocardial function is a major determinant of risk. Patients with low ejection fraction remain at high risk irrespective of the time that has elapsed since the acute infarction.

Prior CABG
Asymptomatic patients within 5 years of successful coronary revascularization are at low risk for perioperative cardiac events.

Prior PCI
Distant (>6 months) PCI should not adversely affect surgery. More recent PCI may be associated with risk for two principal reasons:
- In order to minimize the risk of stent thrombosis, patients usually receive aspirin and clopidogrel (for up to 6 months). The pronounced anti-platelet effect of these drugs poses a risk of haemorrhage and it is preferable to defer surgery until clopidogrel has been stopped for 1 week. When there is active bleeding or major emergency surgery is necessary, platelet transfusion may be given
- Pro-thrombotic conditions associated with surgery can increase the risk of stent thrombosis. Therefore, where possible, it is generally preferred to defer surgery for 4 weeks after stent implantation. This should allow re-endothelialization of the stent without encroaching on the time window for restenosis.

phylactic peri-operative beta-blockade

Jence of the efficacy of peri-operative beta-blockade is mixed. In neral, a patient should continue on beta-blockers for an established ndication (angina, hypertension, arrhythmia). There is some evidence that, particularly in patients undergoing high-risk vascular surgery, pre-treatment with beta blockers may reduce the risk of peri-operative cardiac events. When possible, beta-blockers should be started days or weeks before elective surgery and the dose titrated to obtain a resting heart rate of approximately 60 beats per minute.

Canadian Cardiovascular Society classification of angina

Class I	Symptom free for all normal activities. Angina with strenuous or prolonged effort.
Class II	Minor limitation. Symptoms with brisk effort on stairs, in the cold, or after meals.
Class III	Significant limitation of ordinary activity. Symptoms with one flight of stairs or walking on the flat at a normal pace.
Class IV	Any physical activity may provoke symptoms. Angina at rest.

① Arrhythmias
During anaesthesia and surgery arrhythmias occur frequently and require treatment where there is evidence of haemodynamic compromise (including myocardial ischaemia). See Chapter 9 (📖 p.125)

Arterial hypertension
Hypertension confers a modest increase in the risk of cardiovascular complications of anaesthesia and surgery irrespective of the admission blood pressure. Blood pressure >180/110 requires treatment. However, the presence of target organ involvement is more important than the level of blood pressure.

① Cardiac failure
The patient's functional capacity is useful for predicting operative risk (see NYHA classification 📖 p.75). The ability to climb one flight of stairs with some load (or equivalent) is considered adequate reserve for most surgeries. Heart failure management should be optimized before surgery.

Objective testing
- Echocardiography
- Radionuclide ventriculography (MUGA scan)
- Cardiac magnetic resonance.

Conduction disorders

Pre-operative pacemaker insertion

The indications for pacemaker insertion are covered in Chapter (💷 p.125). The current consensus is that, in general, the indications for pre-operative pacemaker insertion, including temporary pacemaker insertion, are the same as those for the non-surgical setting. These include complete heart block, Mobitz type II block and symptomatic bradycardia.

Valvular heart disease

Considerations relate to (1) haemodynamic consequences (2) anticoagulation (3) risk of endocarditis (4) indirect e.g. arrhythmia, effects of LVH.

See also Chapter 8 on Valve disease 💷 p.90.

Haemodynamic

:**O**: **Severe aortic stenosis** represents the most serious threat. Fixed obstruction to cardiac output permits very little adaptation where increased output is required. Peripheral vasodilatation e.g. from regional anaesthesia or hypotension from haemorrhage cannot be matched by an adequate increase in cardiac output. The consequent fall in blood pressure can lead to coronary hypoperfusion, reduced myocardial function and further hypotension. This is a potentially fatal downward spiral.

ⓘ Even in **moderate aortic stenosis**, stiffness of the left ventricle reduces the tolerance of variability of filling conditions. In fluid overload, the left atrial pressure will increase sharply provoking pulmonary oedema while low filling pressure (hypovolaemia) or low diastolic filling time (high ventricular rates) will decrease cardiac output. Where symptoms or physical signs suggest aortic stenosis, a pre-operative echocardiogram should be obtained.

:**O**: **Mitral stenosis**. The onset of atrial fibrillation or loss of rate control will decrease diastolic filling and bring about a fall in cardiac output with consequent increase in left atrial pressure. This can provoke an abrupt deterioration in functional class and may cause overt pulmonary oedema.

Mitral and aortic regurgitation require careful fluid management and may benefit from afterload reduction e.g. with nitrates and ACE inhibitors.

In some cases it may be appropriate to alleviate valve lesions prior to surgery. Full discussion of valve interventions and their indications are given in Chapter 8 (💷 p.92). In considering intervention, the balance of risk must take into account the type of valve and the possibility of thromboembolic events or infective endocarditis related to future surgery.

agulation (📖 p.109)

echanical prosthetic valves: anticoagulation has to be discontinued
efore most surgeries. Warfarin is replaced by an intravenous infusion
of heparin to facilitate pre- and post-operative anticoagulation
In emergencies, anticoagulation with warfarin can be transiently
reversed by administration of fresh frozen plasma (FFP), which
provides clotting factors

• Be very wary of giving vitamin K since this will prevent anticoagulation
  with warfarin for a prolonged period. With expert guidance, small
  dose of vitamin K (e.g. 1 mg), can be administered.

⑦ Endocarditis avoidance

Abnormal heart valves, prosthetic mechanical valves, or biological valves
are at increased risk for infective endocarditis as organisms are introduced at the time of surgery. Full discussion on the risks of bacteraemia
and on the nature and indications for prophylactic antibiotics are dis-
cussed in Chapter 8 on Valve disease (📖 p.96).

Keep vascular access to the minimum necessary. Take precautions to
avoid infections at insertion. Observe the skin around lines for signs of
infection and revise lines regularly. Seek to remove all vascular catheters
as soon as they are no longer needed.

Pacemakers and implantable defibrillators

Establish the type of pacemaker or defibrillator, the indications for
implantation and the functional settings from the patient's pacemaker
identification card or from the centre where it was implanted. Blindly to
return the pacemaker to its simplest mode of operation by passing a
magnet over it is inadvisable as it is hazardous with modern complex
pacemakers/defibrillators.

These devices are susceptible to electromagnetic interference (EMI).
This can come from disparate sources but in the context of surgery, EMI
from diathermy equipment is the major concern. EMI may enter the
device by direct electrical interference during diathermy or exposure to
an electromagnetic field (device lead acting as aerial). Bipolar leads, generally used in contemporary pacing systems, are much less sensitive to
EMI than unipolar leads. EMI can result in:

• Inappropriate inhibition or triggering of paced output
• Asynchronous pacing
• Reprogramming (usually into a back-up mode)
• Damage to circuitry, or triggering of defibrillator discharge
• Defibrillators may interpret electrocautery as VF and deliver a shock.

Electrocautery is usually applied in unipolar configuration between the
handheld instrument (cathode) and the anode attached to the patient's skin.

• Diathermy should be avoided near the pacemaker/ICD generator
• Bipolar diathermy should be used wherever possible.

Cardiac surgery

The following is intended as a practical guide to situations commonly experienced after cardiac surgery.

Assessing the hypotensive patient post cardiac surgery

Read the operation note and anaesthetic chart. Was the operation straightforward? The surgeon will have noted any difficulties e.g. where small calibre coronary arteries prejudice graft patency or problems with haemostasis. What was the pre-operative assessment of left ventricular function?

Note the blood pressure and pulse trends. Was there an abrupt change suggestive of an acute 'event' or has the change been gradual. Compare with pre-operative values. Determine peripheral perfusion. Is the patient cold and 'shut down' or peripherally vasodilated? What is the urine output?

Is the patient adequately filled? One size does not fit all in this respect. Patients with left ventricular hypertrophy but good LV systolic function (e.g. post aortic valve replacement) are likely to require higher filling pressures. In patients with significant tricuspid regurgitation (e.g. post mitral valve replacement), filling will be difficult to gauge from the venous pressure. Remember that early after surgery, you are likely to have the benefit of a CVP line—🕮 p.11.

Does the ECG show evidence of myocardial ischaemia? Has the rhythm changed? AF is common post-operatively (see opposite). New onset or fast AF may be sufficient to compromise blood pressure in susceptible patients.

Are the pericardial drains productive? Has the rate of drainage changed (new bleeding, drain occlusion)? Hypotension with tachycardia, and elevated CVP may indicate pericardial tamponade. This can occur rapidly and may be caused by a relatively small volume of pericardial blood. Tamponade may embarrass cardiac output due to its effects on filling. Post-operatively, this may be caused by localized effects on a single chamber. An urgent echocardiogram should be obtained. In extreme cases, sudden haemodynamic collapse necessitates emergency exploration and direct drainage with the chest re-opened.

When hypotension persists despite correction of the reversible causes, further evaluation with echocardiography may be indicated. New wall motion abnormalities suggest peri-operative infarction or 'stunning'. Consider support with inotropic drugs ± intra-aortic balloon counterpulsation. These measures are considered in greater detail in the Chapter 1, on Cardiovascular collapse (🕮 p.4).

fibrillation post cardiac surgery

- curs in approximately 25% of patients
- re frequent in elderly patients and those with a prior history of AF
- arkedly compromised patients need DC cardioversion
- Correct hypokalaemia: keep K^+ at 4–5 mmol/L
- Likely to return spontaneously to sinus rhythm, unless AF was present pre-operatively
- Control rate with beta-blocker or digoxin
- Amiodarone IV (central line) may hasten reversion to sinus. In selected patients, continuation with oral therapy may be indicated
- Anticoagulation is needed if persistent (heparin → warfarin)
- Outpatient review of continuing need for antiarrhythmic therapy ± cardioversion.

Atrioventricular conduction block post cardiac surgery

- Most likely after aortic valve surgery because of the valve's proximity to the AV node
- Pacing is necessary using epicardial pacing electrodes implanted at surgery or a temporary transvenous system
- Permanent pacemaker implantation is often required. Predicted by pre-operative features: AV block, LBBB, root abscess, calcified aortic annulus, aortic regurgitation and prior MI.

Post-pericardiotomy syndrome

Inflammatory (possibly autoimmune) pericarditis that occurs >1 week after cardiac surgery where the pericardium has been opened. The associated effusion may be serous or serosanguinous. It can be large and can lead to tamponade. Often associated with fever, pericarditic pain and malaise. The diagnosis is clinical. Echocardiography is helpful in helping to determine the size, distribution, percutaneous accessibility, composition (e.g. fibrinous) and haemodynamic significance of the pericardial effusion. Treat with NSAIDs. Usually self-limiting, but may recur.

Reference

Eagle KA, Berger PB, Calkins H *et al.* (2002). ACC/AHA guideline update for perioperative cardiovascular evaluation for non-cardiac surgery—executive summary. A report of the American College of Cardiology/American Heart Association Task Force on Practice Guidelines. *Circulation* **105**,1257–1267.

Weblink

http://www.acc.org/clinical/guidelines/perio/exec_summ/pdf/periop_execsumm.pdf

Cardiotoxic drug overdose

General approach 262
Cardiac drugs
Beta-blockers 264
Calcium channel blockers 265
Digoxin 266
Non-cardiac drugs
Tricyclic antidepressants 268
Theophylline 269
Drugs used in cancer 270
Recreational drugs
Cocaine 272
Amphetamine 272
Ecstasy 273
Drug-induced QT prolongation 274

General approach

Cardiovascular side-effects can occur with both cardiac and nor
medication. In particular, side-effects secondary to recreational dr
are becoming more prevalent. Patient history may be unreliable an
witnesses should be sought.

▶ This chapter should be used as a brief guide—detailed information
available (see below).

▶ Specialist advice should be sought for overdoses in children.

General management principles
- Resuscitate the patient
- Consider the prevention of drug absorption:
  - Activated charcoal (50 g orally) will absorb many drugs if given
    <1 hour after ingestion
  - Gastric lavage can be considered if a substantial overdose has been
    ingested <1 hour previously. The evidence for benefit is weak and it
    is performed less commonly now
- Supportive care (e.g. airway maintenance, acid-base and electrolyte
  balance, treat seizures) is important
- Any unstable arrhythmias (VT, fast SVT >180/min) are better dealt
  with by cardioversion than drugs.

Sources of information
TOXBASE—web-based service accessible from any emergency dept.
http://www.spib.axl.co.uk

In the United Kingdom, the **Poisons Information Service 0870 6006266**—
directs callers to local unit.

① Beta-blockers

Clinical features

- Light-headedness, dizziness, syncope
- Bradycardia
- Hypotension
- Heart failure (esp. if pre-existing LV dysfunction)
- Drowsiness, confusion, convulsions
- Cardiorespiratory arrest, due to asystole or VF (rare)
- Bronchospasm (uncommon).

Investigations

ECG: AV block, intraventricular conduction defects (RBBB, LBBB), ventricular extrasystoles, asystole.

Management

- Consider activated charcoal (or lavage for substantial overdoses) if <1 hr
- Observe for at least 6 hrs (12 hrs if slow-release preparation)
- *Atropine* for symptomatic bradycardia & hypotension (3 mg IV bolus)
- *IV fluids* for hypotension
- *Glucagon* for severe bradycardia, hypotension or heart failure unresponsive to atropine; increases myocardial cAMP, thereby acting as an inotrope; (2–10 mg IV bolus followed, if necessary, by IV infusion 1–5 mg/hr). Can cause vomiting, so anti-emetic sometimes required
- *Pacing:* Temporary transvenous or external pacing should be considered if atropine and glucagon are ineffective (📖 p.296)
- *Salbutamol* for bronchospasm (5–10 mg nebulized)
- *Dextrose:* If hypoglycaemia develops, give 25 mL of 50% dextrose. Monitor blood glucose closely
- *Inotropes:* In severe cases, may be needed to maintain cardiac output e.g. dobutamine (2.5–10 µg/kg/min) or isoprenaline (5–10 µg/min) by IV infusion.

▶ Sotalol has additional class III anti-arrhythmic action and can cause QT prolongation and Torsade de Pointes (📖 p.274).

▶ Prognosis is worsened in those taking concomitant calcium-channel blocker therapy.

alcium channel blockers

cal features

- ausea, vomiting, dizziness
- lurred speech, confusion, convulsion
- Hypotension
- Hyperglycaemia, metabolic acidosis.

Dihydropyridine group (e.g. nifedipine, amlodipine):
- Sinus tachycardia.

Non-dihydropyridine group (e.g. diltiazem, verapamil):
- Sinus bradycardia, AV block
- ↓myocardial contractility, pulmonary oedema.

Investigations

ECG: as for beta-blockers.

Management

- Consider activated charcoal or gastric lavage (📖 p.262). Sustained release preparations may require further charcoal every 4 hours, plus a single dose of osmotic laxative (e.g. lactulose, MgSO₄)
- Monitor for ≥4 hours (≥12 hours if sustained-release preparation)
- *Calcium chloride* (0.2 mL/kg of 10% solution, up to 10 mL, IV over 5 min) for significant clinical features (or *calcium gluconate* at 2–3 times dose). Can be repeated every 10–20 min up to 4 doses. May reverse prolonged intracardiac conduction times
- *Glucagon* for severe myocardial depression or hypotension. (1 mg IV every 3 min). Consider infusion (2–4 mg/hr) if good response
- Consider atropine, pacing and inotropes as for beta-blockers.

▶ Prognosis is worsened in those taking concomitant beta-blocker therapy.

① Digoxin

Chronic toxicity may be as a result of interactions with other albu~~
bound drugs (e.g. amiodarone) or from progressive renal failure. Dig~~
has a long half-life (16–20 hours); the half-life of digitoxin (a related co~~
pound) is 6 days.

Toxicity is more common following acute overdosage if already on
digoxin or cardiovascular disease is present.

Clinical features
- Nausea and vomiting
- Dizziness, slurred speech, confusion, visual disturbances (blurring, alteration in colour perception), and hallucinations
- Hyperkalaemia
- Arrhythmias, hypotension, cardiac arrest
- Life-threatening toxicity rare in healthy hearts if <5 mg ingested. Those with cardiac disease are much more susceptible.

Investigations

ECG
Marked sinus bradycardia, PR and QRS prolongation, sinus arrest, supraventricular arrhythmias, AV block, ventricular ectopics, VT, VF. A classical arrhythmia in chronic toxicity is paroxysmal atrial tachycardia with AV block.

Blood
- Serum digoxin level—immediate if acute overdose and severe toxicity present (digoxin antibodies being considered). Otherwise wait >6 hours post-dose. Normal therapeutic range 0.8–2.0 mg/L
- Serum electrolytes (esp. K^+)
- Magnesium.

Management
- Consider activated charcoal if <1 hour from ingestion
- Monitor for at least 6 hours
- Cardiac monitoring and frequent BP measurement
- Treat hyperkalaemia aggressively (but avoid calcium gluconate as it may precipitate VF)
- Correct hypokalaemia with oral or IV K^+ supplementation
- *Atropine:* for symptomatic bradycardia and AV block (1–2 mg IV)
- *Lidocaine, β-blocker or amiodarone* for VT
- *Pacing* if severe bradycardia/sinus arrest
- *Digoxin-specific Ab (Digibind ®):* Given in severe cases if K^+>5.5 mmol/L or a satisfactory cardiac output is not achieved in patients with sinus arrest, AV block, severe bradycardia or tachyarrhythmias. Patients usually respond within 1 hour. Cardiac monitoring required for 24 hours; can cause ↓K^+, so monitor K^+ frequently. See box for dose.

...d® dosage for toxicity during chronic therapy

..dult patients in whom the steady-state digoxin level is known:

$$\text{Number of vials} = \frac{\text{Serum digoxin conc. (ng/mL)} \times \text{weight (kg)}}{100}$$

- In adult patients in whom the steady-state digoxin level is unknown, 6 vials of Digibind® (228 mg) usually reverses toxicity.

Digibind® dosage for acute poisoning

- Methods for calculating dose are usually by an estimate of the amount of digoxin ingested in milligrams (*not* micrograms):

$$\text{Number of vials} = \frac{\text{Total dose ingested (mg)} \times 0.8}{0.5 \text{ (mg of digitalis bound per vial)}}$$

- 20 vials of Digibind® (760 mg) usually reverses acute toxicity if the amount ingested is unknown.

Predisposing factors for digoxin toxicity
- Acute hypoxia
- Electrolyte disturbance, esp. ↓K^+
- Respiratory alkalosis
- Myocardial ischaemia
- Old age
- Drug interactions
- Impaired renal/hepatic clearance.

Poor prognostic indicators
- Older patients
- Underlying cardiac disease
- Hyperkalaemia (>5 mmol/L)
- High grade AV block
- Serum digoxin level >15 ng/mL
- VT.

① Tricyclic antidepressants

Clinical features

- Anticholinergic: dry mouth, blurred vision, urinary retention
- Palpitation, supraventricular and ventricular arrhythmias
- Hyper-reflexia, extensor plantar responses
- Syncope, convulsions, absent brain-stem reflexes in severe cases.

Investigations

ECG

- Sinus tachycardia, ↓P wave amplitude, prolonged PR interval
- QRS prolongation (>100 msec: significant intoxication, >160 msec generally seen before ventricular arrhythmias occur)
- Supraventricular and ventricular arrhythmias (usually <6 hrs).

Blood

Arterial blood gas (metabolic acidosis), U&E.

Management

- Supportive measures including IV fluids ± inotropes
- Activated charcoal: if ingestion < 1 hr previously
- Sodium bicarbonate alters myocardial binding of tricyclics: give 50 mmol (350 mL of 1.26% or 50 mL of 8.4% (the latter through a central line)) over 20 mins if any of:
  - pH <7.1
  - QRS duration >160 msec (even in the absence of acidosis)
  - Arrhythmias
  - Significant hypotension
- In general, antiarrhythmic drugs should be avoided and aggressive measures to correct the underlying metabolic and clinical state (hypoxia, hypotension, acidosis, ↓K⁺) should be pursued instead
- IV diazepam for convulsions. ⚠ Phenytoin is contraindicated.

Theophylline

Clinical features

- Agitation, tremor, drowsiness, convulsions, status epilepticus
- Hypokalaemia, acidosis
- Sinus tachycardia, hypotension, SVT, VT, VF.

Investigations

ECG: Sinus tachycardia, SVT, VT, VF.
Blood: U&E (esp. K^+), Mg^{2+}, arterial blood gases, theophylline levels.

Management

- Consider activated charcoal. Repeat doses every 4 hrs if plasma theophylline >40 mg/L
- Monitor vital signs. Cardiac monitoring for >4 hrs
- Check K^+ and blood gases regularly—initial K^+ may not reflect total K^+ depletion; additionally, rebound hyperkalaemia may occur during recovery. In severe poisoning, measure 1–2 hrly
- IV fluids ± inotropes for hypotension
- Benzodiazepines or phenytoin for convulsions
- Beta-blockers or verapamil for symptomatic or compromising SVT (asymptomatic can be left untreated)
- VT: synchronized DC cardioversion (📖 p.302) or magnesium sulphate
- In very severe cases, haemodialysis may be required.

Drugs used in cancer

A number of oncological therapeutic agents are known to be cardiotoxic. In the majority, these effects are cumulative, but a number of medications have acute cardiac side-effects:

① *Interleukin-2*
- Causes a capillary leak syndrome (hypotension, oedema, effusions, arrhythmias)
- Stop infusion, administer steroids, antihistamines and consider epinephrine.

① *5-Fluorouracil*
- May cause myocardial ischaemia and acute MI
- Stop 5-FU treatment and treat with conventional anti-anginal therapy.

⑦ *Anthracyclines* e.g. *doxorubicin, daunorubicin*
- Chronic dose-related cardiomyopathy
- Arrhythmias.

Others
Cisplatin	Acute myocardial ischaemia
Cyclophosphamide	Heart failure, haemorrhagic pericarditis
Mitomycin C	Myocardial injury
Vincristine	MI
Vinblastine	MI
Taxol	Bradycardia.

Cocaine

Clinical features
- Euphoria, agitation, paranoia
- Sweating, hyperthermia, convulsions
- Tachycardia, hypertension, chest pain, pulmonary oedema
- Coronary/carotid spasm—can be severe enough to cause MI/stroke
- Intracerebral haemorrhage
- The patient may be violent and have a high pain threshold.

Investigations
ECG: ST segment elevation/depression if coronary ischaemia, supraventricular and ventricular arrhythmias.
Blood: U&E, cardiac enzymes, arterial blood gases.

Management
- ① Cooling (tepid sponging, chilled IV fluids) if core temperature >41°C, aiming for <39°C
- Diazemuls to control agitation or convulsions (5–10 mg IV)
- ① Nitrates may relieve myocardial ischaemia and lower blood pressure (e.g. GTN 1–10 mg/kg/hr IV infusion)
- Adenosine (6–18 mg IV) or verapamil (5 mg IV) for sustained, haemodynamically tolerated SVTs
- Phentolamine for hypertension and coronary spasm (2–5 mg IV bolus)
- ⚙: Thrombolysis should be considered if persistent ST segment elevation is present and there are no contraindications (consider primary angioplasty if contraindications present)
- ⚙: Broad complex tachycardia can be treated with sodium bicarbonate (📖 p.268).

▶ Beta-blockers should be avoided as they may be associated with unopposed alpha-receptor-mediated vasoconstriction, which can result in a sudden and severe increase in blood pressure and coronary vasoconstriction.

Amphetamine

The cardiological features and management of amphetamine overdose are comparable to those of cocaine overdose (see above).

...asy

(...nethylene-dioxy-methamphetamine or MDMA)

...inical features
- Nausea, muscle pain, hyperthermia, ataxia, rhabdomyolysis
- Euphoria, agitation
- Hyper/hypotension, tachyarrhythmias
- Hyponatraemia, hyperkalaemia, ARDS.

Investigations
ECG: Sinus tachycardia or SVT.
Blood: U&E (esp. Na$^+$), liver function tests, arterial blood gases.

Management
- Cooling: To reduce core body temperature to <39°C (e.g. tepid sponging, chilled IV fluids). Consider dantrolene (1mg/kg IV over 15 mins)
- Beta-blocker to treat narrow complex tachycardia (e.g. metoprolol 5–10 mg IV)
- Hypertension—Diazemuls® and/or nitrates IV.

Drug-induced QT prolongation

Many factors influence acquired QT prolongation, including genetic sceptibility (separate from congenital long-QT syndromes), metab state (including hypokalaemia and hypomagnesaemia), other concomita drugs, and heart rate. Thus the emergence of QT prolongation relies not just on the drug ingested, but on a combination of this and many predisposing factors. The occurrence with any particular drug is therefore unpredictable, but several drugs have been shown to be associated:

▶ The main risk is of polymorphic VT (Torsade de Pointes) (📖 p.160).

Some causative drugs	
Class 1a antiarrhythmics:	Quinidine, procainamide, disopyramide
Class 1c antiarrhythmics:	Flecainide
Class III antiarrhythmics:	Sotalol, amiodarone, dofetilide
Tricyclic antidepressants:	Amitryptiline, imipramine, clomipramine
Psychotropic agents:	Lithium, chlorpromazine, haloperidol
Antihistamines:	Terfenadine, loratidine
Antimicrobials:	Erythromycin, clarithromycin, quinine, chloroquine, ketoconazole
Immunosuppressants:	Tacrolimus
Recreational drugs:	Cocaine.

Clinical features
- Recurrent dizziness or syncope
- Palpitations
- Polymorphic ventricular tachycardia/Torsade de Pointes.

Investigations
ECG: VT, Torsade de Pointes.
Blood: Serum electrolytes (esp. K^+, Mg^{2+}, Ca^{2+}).

Management
- Identify and withdrawing the offending drug(s)
- Avoid empirical antiarrhythmic therapy
- For Torsade:
  - Mg^{2+} 8 mmol of $MgSO_4$ over 15 minutes, then 72 mmol over 24 hrs
  - K^+ Keep at 4.5–5 mmol/L
  - Pacing Overdrive pacing for VT—rate higher than the VT— (📖 p.161), or prevention of VT in bradycardia with long QT.

▶ Concurrent use of agents that prolong QT interval and/or inhibit hepatic cytochrome P450 isoenzyme (e.g. fluoxetine) should be avoided.

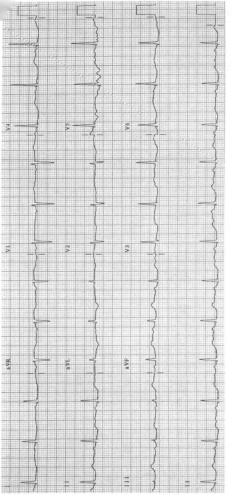

Drug induced long QT .

Miscellaneous conditions

Hypertensive emergencies *278*
Traumatic heart disease *280*
Cardiac tumours *282*

⊙ Hypertensive emergencies

A *hypertensive crisis* (previously called 'malignant hypertension') occ
<1% of patients with hypertension. Severe prolonged elevation of b
pressure (diastolic >130 mmHg) can result in end-organ damage, mos
affecting the central nervous system, kidneys and cardiovascular system.
Prognosis depends on the degree of end-organ damage, rather than the
level of the blood pressure. Survival rate has improved considerably and
>90% of patients are alive at 1 year.

Presentation
- Angina, left ventricular failure
- Headache, visual disturbance, irritability, altered consciousness,
  seizures (hypertensive encephalopathy)
- Nausea and vomiting
- In the setting of aortic dissection
- Haematuria or acute renal failure
- In association with catecholamine excess (phaeochromocytoma,
  recreational drug overdose)
- During pregnancy with eclampsia/pre-eclampsia.

Clinical signs
- Check blood pressure in both arms (?aortic dissection) and in the legs
  (?coarctation)
- Fundoscopy (retinal haemorrhages, exudates, or papilloedema)
- Full neurological examination (focal abnormalities)
- Examine for renal bruits (?renal artery stenosis).

Investigations
- 12 lead ECG
- Chest X-ray
- FBC (microangiopathic haemolytic anaemia), U&E, glucose, clotting
  studies (disseminated intravascular coagulation)
- Urinalysis
- Further laboratory investigations (according to working diagnosis)
  include cardiac troponin, thyroid hormones, urine collections for
  catecholamines.

Management
- Patients are usually admitted to hospital for bed rest and monitoring
- Initial aim of blood pressure management is to lower systolic pressure
  by 10% in the first hour and then by a further 15% in the next few
  hours
- Treatment can usually be commenced orally with a beta-blocker
  (e.g. atenolol) or long acting calcium antagonist (e.g. amlodipine)
- IV antihypertensive therapy may be required if oral therapy is not
  effective—e.g. nitrates, nitroprusside, labetalol (📖 p.174).

...nsive emergencies in specific conditions

    dissection (📖 p.170). A more rapid reduction in blood pressure
    ...quired with a target systolic pressure of <120 mmHg
    ...ients with *subarachnoid haemorrhage* should be considered for
    ...eatment with nimodipine intravenously (0.5–2 mg/hour via central
    ...ine) or orally (60 mg every 4 hours)
- Patients with *phaeochromocytoma* should be considered for initial
  treatment with the alpha-blocker phentolamine (2–5 mg intravenously)
  followed by beta-blockade if necessary. The risk of beta-blockade is of
  unopposed alpha-adrenoreceptor stimulation
- In *pregnancy* some anti-hypertensive drugs are contraindicated.
  📖 p.214 for specific advice
- *Cocaine* abuse may precipitate a hypertensive emergency (📖 p.272).
  Intravenous benzodiazepines and vasodilator therapy are
  recommended
- Hypertension caused by *monoamine oxidase inhibitors* should be
  managed with benzodiazepines and with a short acting antihypertensive
  such as sodium nitroprusside.

Further management
A combination of beta-blockers, calcium channel blockers, ACE-inhibitors
and other antihypertensives are often necessary to normalize blood
pressure.

Traumatic heart disease

① Blunt cardiac trauma

- Usually occurs as a result of motor vehicle accidents, crush injuries, falls, prolonged cardiopulmonary resuscitation
- Injuries range from myocardial bruising to fatal cardiac rupture
- Non-fatal injury usually results in sub-epicardial or myocardial bruising
- Investigations for blunt cardiac trauma include:
  - ECG—T wave changes (non-specific) or conduction abnormalities (bundle branch block)
  - Cardiac enzymes can be elevated (though not believed to be prognostically important)
  - Echocardiography may show regional wall motion abnormalities or a pericardial effusion
- Management is bed rest, monitoring, and analgesia
- Complete recovery is the rule.

Commotio cordis

A cause of sudden cardiac death, particularly in young men with no underlying cardiac disease. Impact to the precordium (usually from a baseball or other hard object) over the centre of the left ventricle just before the onset of the T wave is believed to cause VF and sudden death.

⚙: Penetrating cardiac trauma

▶▶ Refer immediately to a cardiothoracic surgeon.

- Stab and gunshot wounds are the commonest causes and usually affect the right and left ventricles (anterior structures)
- A large proportion of stab wounds to the heart present with pericardial tamponade whereas gun shot victims usually present with shock due to haemorrhage
- Immediate ultrasonography is indicated and if a pericardial effusion is visible in an unstable patient, urgent cardiothoracic intervention is required
- Pericardiocentesis is discouraged in acute trauma. The blood clots quickly and may be difficult to remove
- Do not remove a knife or other penetrating instrument unless instructed to do so by a cardiothoracic surgeon.

⑦ Cardiac tumours

Primary cardiac tumours are rare. Secondary malignant deposits in t.
heart are more common. Three-quarters of primary cardiac tumours
are benign and the majority of these are myxomas. Diagnosis is by echocardiography, MRI, and CT imaging.

Clinical features

- Cardiac symptoms and signs related to obstruction (dyspnoea from
  pulmonary venous congestion and pulmonary oedema, syncope)
- Signs of systemic embolization (stroke, peripheral emboli 🕮 p.202)
- Systemic or constitutional symptoms (fever, weight loss, fatigue)
- Arrhythmias (due to direct infiltration of the conduction tissue or
  myocardial irritation).

▶ Cardiac tumours are the great mimickers.

Benign tumours

Cardiac myxomas

Represent 50% of cardiac tumours. Rare forms are multiple (LAMB and
NAME syndromes) and inherited (autosomal dominant). Usually present
around age 50. Most commonly arise in the atria from the fossa ovalis.
Left atrium > right atrium. Symptoms and signs (clubbing, rash, 'tumour
plop'—similar to 3rd heart sound) similar to endocarditis, malignancy and
collagen vascular disease. Blood test may reveal anaemia, ↑CRP, ↑ESR.
Echocardiography is normally diagnostic (see opposite). Myxomas generally have a broad base but some are pedicled. Management is urgent
surgical excision. Follow-up echocardiography is required as inadequate
excision can lead to recurrence.

Papillary fibroelastomas

Often detected as small incidental lesions on the aortic and mitral valve.
Fragments may embolize leading to coronary or cerebral obstruction.
Surgery is generally indicated to improve prognosis but small right sided
lesions may be monitored.

Others

- Rhabdomyoma (most common primary cardiac neoplasm in children)
- Fibroma (most commonly resected childhood tumour)
- Haemangiomas
- Cardiac lipomas
- AV nodal tumours (small cystic mass—a cause of sudden cardiac
  death).

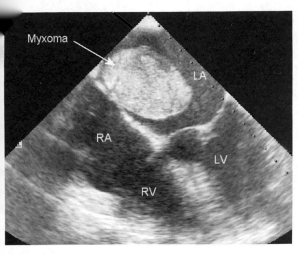

Transoesophageal echocardiography demonstrating a large myxoma attached to the septum between the right atrium (RA) and left atrium (LA).

Malignant tumours

Sarcomas
Extremely rare. May occur in any part of the heart but most commonly involve the right atrium. Includes angiosarcoma, osteosarcoma, leiomyosarcoma, rhabdomyosarcoma. Management is with a combination of surgery, chemotherapy and radiotherapy. Outcome is generally poor with median survival <1 year.

Cardiac lymphoma
Radiological staging is required to distinguish between primary cardiac lymphoma and generalized lymphoma. Management is usually with chemotherapy.

Metastatic cardiac tumour
Tachycardia, arrhythmias, heart failure in a patient with carcinoma should raise the suspicion. May present with pericardial effusion and/or tamponade. Associated malignancies include malignant melanoma, leukaemia, lymphoma, carcinoma of the stomach, liver, colon, rectum, and ovary.

Practical issues

Practical procedures

General considerations 288
Central venous lines 290
Pulmonary artery (PA) catheters 294
Temporary pacing 296
Inserting an arterial line 298
Pericardiocentesis 300
Cardioversion/defibrillation 302

General considerations

There is always time to think

There are very few emergencies that require an *immediate* response. A focused period of reflection and planning, supported when required by the opinion and contribution of others is an essential prelude to the successful performance of a practical procedure—especially in the demanding setting of an acute clinical problem.

▶ Is the proposed procedure indicated?

This may seem an odd first question but it is the correct starting point. Many a practical procedure is abandoned after prolonged or multiple fruitless (and often painful) attempts with an observation to the patient that 'We can do without it'. Consider the indications for the proposed procedure and any special factors that may affect the likelihood of success or the objective risk. Review all alternative approaches to the problem. Commit to a procedure only if the intervention is considered essential or has much to offer, at a risk judged acceptable to your patient. A process of informed consent is ideal but may not be possible or appropriate in certain clinical settings.

▶ Do you have the skills to perform the procedure?

To thine own self be true. It is your professional duty to act within the bounds of your established competence. Never hesitate to ask for help or guidance or to initiate a referral to an appropriate specialist. This text aspires to serve as a practical *aide-memoire* and is not a substitute for formal training and practical experience. Even if experienced and confident in a procedure, never underestimate the role and importance of assistants or other professionals (e.g. radiographers in temporary pacing).

▶ Do you have the setting and equipment for the procedure?

Remember the rule of the 13 Ps:
In the Performance of Practical Procedures, Proper Prior Preparation and Planning and Perfect Patient Positioning, Prevent Poor Performance.
- If appropriate, inform your senior cover of your intention and schedule
- Secure time, free of likely interruption
  - Who will hold your bleep?
  - Are there any competing urgent clinical concerns?
- Rearrange the room and furniture to secure optimum access
  - Adjust patient position, bed height and remove obstructions
- Ensure adequate lighting
- Prepare and check all items of equipment that will be required
- For complex or unfamiliar procedures, perform a mental rehearsal
  - To establish the sequence of your planned action
  - To checklist all planned equipment requirements
- Ensure compatibility of interdependent items
  - Will the pacing wire fit through the venous access line?
  - Will the pacing wire fit to the pacing box?
- Prepare in advance items that do not demand sterile handling e.g.
  - Infusions for central venous lines
  - Transducers and monitors for pressure lines.

Central venous lines

Choice of approach

The three main approaches to central venous cannulation are:
(1) internal jugular vein, (2) subclavian vein, and (3) femoral vein.
You should aim to become familiar with at least two of these routes.

General points—applicable to all approaches

- Pay attention to sterility to minimise infection risk. Prepare the skin and drape with sterile dressings. Wear sterile gloves and a gown
- The patient should be positioned with head-down tilt. This fills the central veins, increasing their available size for cannulation and minimizes the risk of air embolization during the procedure
- Whenever possible use the Seldinger (guidewire through needle) technique. Catheter over needle devices (similar to peripheral IV cannulae) are more difficult to place
- Mount the needle on a syringe containing a few mL of 0.9% saline
- Position the guidewire on the sterile field but within easy reach
- Advance the needle, maintaining negative pressure by aspiration
- If the vein is not entered, withdraw the needle slowly maintaining syringe aspiration. Sometimes the needle transfixes the vein and cannulation is only evident on slow withdrawal
- After an unsuccessful pass:
  - Flush the needle to remove debris that may clog its lumen
  - Reassess the anatomical landmarks and identify a modified line for the next attempt. Explore the region systematically
- When the needle enters the vein and blood is aspirated, be prepared to make minor adjustments (advance or retract) to ensure free flow of blood
- Fix the needle with one hand and carefully remove the syringe
- Pass the flexible end of the guidewire down the needle. The wire should pass with minimal resistance. Passage can sometimes be facilitated with minor rotation of the wire or needle (to change the angle of the bevel)
- If resistance persists remove the wire and check the needle position by aspiration with a syringe
- When half of the wire is in the vein, remove the needle and place the cannula and its dilator over the wire. Do not advance the sheath into the body until a short length of wire is visible protruding from the distal end of the dilator and is secured with a firm grasp
- If there is resistance to insertion of the cannula, consider enlarging the skin nick. If there is resistance in the deeper layers (e.g. clavipectoral fascia for subclavian lines) it may be necessary to first advance a dilator of smaller caliber (without its sheath) to open the track
- Once the line is in place remove the dilator and secure the cannula with suture and a transparent occlusive dressing
- Radiographic examination (penetrated films) can be used to check the line position but this investigation should not preclude emergency use of a line following uncomplicated insertion.

...al jugular (IJ) approach

...has emerged as the most common route for central venous access.
...hen compared to subclavian access, the IJ approach has a reduced risk
of pneumothorax and allows compression haemostasis if bleeding occurs.
The line, once placed may be more uncomfortable for patients and there
may be an increased tendency for displacement of temporary pacing
wires introduced via this access. The right IJ is preferred to the left as it
avoids the thoracic duct.

- Prepare and drape the skin
- Identify the apex of the triangle between the clavicular and manubrial
  heads of sternomastoid (see figure below)
- Infiltrate the skin and subcutaneous tissue with lidocaine 1–2%
- Nick the skin with a small (e.g. Number 11) scalpel blade
- Palpate the line of the carotid artery and insert the needle lateral to
  this line at an angle of 45° to the skin, aiming for the right nipple area
  (or anterior superior iliac spine)
- The vein is superficial and cannulation should be achieved at a depth of
  a few centimeters. Do not advance beyond this as the apex of the lung
  could be injured.

Internal jugular central line insertion

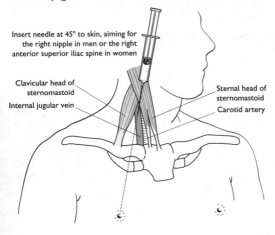

Insert needle at 45° to skin, aiming for the right nipple in men or the right anterior superior iliac spine in women

Clavicular head of sternomastoid

Internal jugular vein

Sternal head of sternomastoid

Carotid artery

Subclavian approach

The subclavian approach allows access to the patient if the area around the patient's head is unavailable (for example during a cardiac arrest). A line inserted by this route lies on the anterior chest, is comfortable for the patient and easy to manage. The main limitations of the approach are a risk of pneumothorax and an inability to apply pressure to the target vessels in the event of multiple venous or inadvertent arterial puncture.

- Prepare and drape the skin
- Identify the junction between the medial third and lateral two-thirds of the clavicle. This is usually at the apex of a convex angulation as the clavicle sweeps laterally and cranially
- The skin incision point is 2 cm inferior and lateral to this point
- Infiltrate the skin and subcutaneous tissue at this point and up to the edge of the clavicle at the first landmark
- Move the needletip stepwise down the clavicle infiltrating local anesthetic. Keep the needle horizontal until it moves below the clavicle
- Prepare the cannulation needle and follow the same initial track as the anesthetic needle
- When the needle lies just below the clavicle swing the needle round to aim at the nadir of the suprasternal notch
- Keeping the needle horizontal and parallel to the bed (avoiding lifting the hands off the body and angling the needle tip down) minimizes the risk of pneumothorax.

Right subclavian vein central line insertion

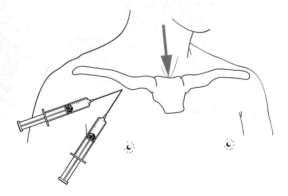

...l vein approach

...noral approach allows easy cannulation of a great vein and is valu-
...n an emergency setting. The area can be compressed in the event of
...eding and temporary pacing can be achieved by this route. The main
...nitations relate to subsequent patient immobility and a probable increased
risk of line infection.

- The patient should be lying flat with the leg slightly adducted and
  externally rotated
- Shave the groin, prepare the skin, and drape
- Palpate the femoral artery below the inguinal ligament, over or
  slightly above the natural skin crease at the top of the leg
- The femoral vein lies medial to the femoral artery
- Infiltrate local anaesthetic at the skin surface and deeper layers
- Advance the cannulation needle at 30–45° to the skin surface
- The vein usually lies ~ 2–4 cm from the skin surface.

Right femoral vein anatomy

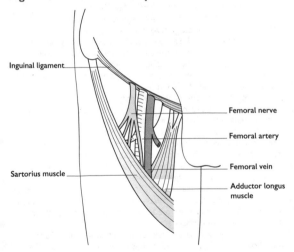

Inguinal ligament

Femoral nerve

Femoral artery

Femoral vein

Sartorius muscle

Adductor longus
muscle

Pulmonary artery (PA) catheters

The main purpose of PA (e.g. Swan–Ganz) catheters is to monitor intrac. pressures. Other, more specialised, catheters allow the calculation of in. of cardiac function and vascular resistance. Ensure that the correct equipme. is available and prepared including the pressure transducers and monitors.

- Connect the patient to ECG monitoring and insert a peripheral IV cannula
- Secure central venous access using a sheath designed to allow the introduction of PA catheters
- Prepare the PA catheter by flushing the lumens—usually labelled distal, mid and proximal, describing the exit lumen in the catheter. Most PA catheters include a soft balloon, inflated with air and designed to encourage floatation of the catheter tip (with blood flow), through the right heart and into the pulmonary vasculature. Test this balloon with an inflation/deflation cycle
- Attach real time pressure monitoring to the distal channel of the PA catheter and insert the catheter to a depth of 8–10 cm
- Inflate the balloon to encourage flow through the right heart. Deep inspiration can encourage passage across the tricuspid valve
- Progress of the catheter can be assessed with X-ray screening but the more usual method is to observe the characteristic waveforms (see figure opposite) recorded in the right atrium, ventricle and in the pulmonary artery. The right ventricle is usually gained at a catheter length of 25–35 cm and the PA at 40–50 cm
- Ventricular ectopics and non-sustained VT may occur during passage (usually indicating that the catheter is in the right ventricle) but do not demand treatment in the absence of circulatory collapse
- Do not continue to advance the catheter if there is no progress. This risks knot formation with catheter coiling in a chamber. Deflate the balloon, withdraw to the right atrium and attempt another passage. In patients with low cardiac output or established right heart pathology specialist help with X-ray imaging may be required
- When in the pulmonary circulation, advance the catheter tip to a position where the wedge pressure can be measured when the balloon is inflated. Deflation of the balloon between readings minimizes the risk of trauma or rupture of a pulmonary vessel
- A good wedge tracing exhibits a classic left atrial pattern with 'a' and 'v' wave morphology (see figure opposite). It is lower or equal to the PA diastolic pressure and has no dichrotic notch (seen in most PA tracings). The wedge pressure usually fluctuates with respiration. If the pressure tracing is damped and tends to increase in a ramp fashion this implies 'overwedging' and partial balloon deflation or catheter withdrawal may be required.

art pressure tracings

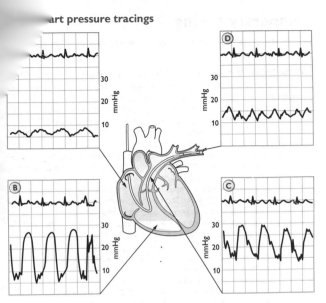

Right heart catheterization. In each panel, the ECG is shown at the top with the corresponding pressure trace from the distal port of a PA catheter at the bottom. The characteristic pressure traces indicate the position of the catheter as it traverses the right heart. Record the pressures obtained from each location and the systemic arterial blood pressure.

A: Right atrial pressure trace in sinus rhythm. Atrial pressure is clearly lower than that of RV or PA. The 'a' wave coincides with atrial contraction while the 'v' wave reflects atrial filling against the tricuspid valve (closed during RV systole). The 'a' wave will be absent in atrial fibrillation. Large 'v' waves are indicative of tricuspid incompetence.

B: The right ventricular pressure trace is characterized by large swings in pressure that correspond to RV contraction and relaxation.

C: In the PA, the systolic should be equal to RV systolic (in the absence of right ventricular outflow tract obstruction or pulmonary stenosis). Note the dicrotic notch corresponding to closure of the pulmonary valve.

D: Pulmonary capillary wedge pressure. With the PA catheter balloon inflated, the distal port is insulated from the right heart and it is effectively exposed to left atrial pressure. In the absence of pulmonary embolism or pre-capillary pulmonary hypertension then PA diastolic pressure should approximate closely to PCWP.

Normal ranges		
RA	0–8 mmHg	
RV	systolic 20–25 mmHg	diastolic 6–12 mmHg
PA	systolic 20–25 mmHg	diastolic 4–8 mmHg
PCWP	6–12 mmHg	

Temporary pacing

▶ Consider drugs or external pacing as a means of immediate s⌐ required.

Transvenous temporary pacemaker insertion

- Insert a peripheral IV cannula and connect an ECG monitor (avoid external wires that will be visible when screening with X-rays)
- Using full sterile precautions, secure central venous access with a sheath of larger diameter than the temporary wire to be used. If subsequent permanent pacing is a possibility, try to leave at least one subclavian venous access untouched
- Under X-ray screening advance the wire into the right atrium. The wire has a J-shaped distal contour which allows the tip to be directed by rotation of the proximal end of the wire
- Direct the wire towards the apex of the right ventricle (this lies just medial to the apex of the cardiac silhouette on AP screening)
- If the wire does not move directly over the tricuspid valve it may be necessary to form a loop of wire in the atrium, usually achieved with the tip on the right lateral atrial border. Rotation and advancement of the wire may then result in prolapse through the tricuspid valve
- As the wire enters the ventricle some ectopic activity is usual and helps confirm a ventricular position
- The wire can inadvertently enter the coronary sinus. Its orifice lies above the tricuspid valve. A wire in the coronary sinus appears more cranial on AP screening and on a lateral view moves posterior (rather than the desired anterior direction of a right ventricular lead)
- Manipulate the wire so that the tip curves downwards to the apex of the ventricle. In its final position the line of the wire should resemble the heel of a sock in the right atrium (see figure), with the toe in the apex of the right ventricle
- Connect the lead to the pacing box and test the threshold for capture. Pace at a rate above the intrinsic cardiac rate while slowly turning down the box output (start at 3 V). The ECG monitor is observed to identify the output at which capture is lost. Increase again slowly to recapture. This is the pacing threshold. A threshold of ≤1 V is desirable. Output is set to at least 3× the pacing threshold
- Test the stability of the lead position by observing lead motion and the ability to pace the heart during deep inspiration and coughing
- Suture the lead and sheath to the skin and apply transparent occlusive dressings
- Secure the external portion of the lead with tape or other fixatives. Fixing a loop on the skin should mean that inadvertent tugs on the wire will tighten the loop rather than pulling out the wire.

External (transcutaneous) temporary pacing

With gel pads at apex and right parasternal position, set rate to 70/min in demand mode. Turn up output until electrical capture and confirm output with pulse. Note uncomfortable skeletal muscle contraction will occur and may result in ECG artifact. Sedation usually required.

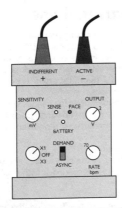

Configuring the pacemaker settings

Set to DEMAND at a RATE of e.g. 70 beats per minute. The pacemaker will, on a beat to beat basis, PACE when it does not detect ventricular activity above that rate. The red PACE light will illuminate on each occasion. When the spontaneous ventricular rate is above the pacemaker rate, the box will inhibit and the red SENSE light will illuminate. An OUTPUT set to at least 3× pacemaker threshold will ensure that each impulse 'captures' the ventricle. The SENSITIVITY should be adjusted to ensure that each intrinsic beat is detected but that skeletal muscle interference does not lead to pacemaker inhibition (the lower the setting, the more sensitive the pacemaker).
❶ Note that instigating pacing may lead to pacemaker dependence.
❶ Ensure that the pacemaker is set to DEMAND. Asynchronous pacing risks inducing ventricular arrhythmias.

Temporary pacing wire position

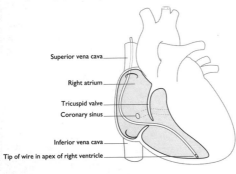

Superior vena cava

Right atrium

Tricuspid valve
Coronary sinus

Inferior vena cava

Tip of wire in apex of right ventricle

Inserting an arterial line

Although the femoral and brachial arteries can be used, the best app[...]
is via the radial artery. This is a superficial vessel, easily palpated at the [...]
medial to the radial styloid. In the vast majority of people, a dual bl[...]
supply to the hand (via the ulnar artery and palmar arch) ensures adequa[...]
distal limb perfusion even if the radial artery is occupied by a catheter o[...]
closes by subsequent thrombosis.

• Revise the general considerations for venous line insertion (💭 p.290)
• Position the patient's hand palm upwards. Place a support (bandage
  roll or 500 mL fluid bag) to support the lower forearm and allow the
  wrist to rest in passive extension
• Prepare and drape the wrist
• Infiltrate local anaesthetic at the skin surface and subcutaneous layer
• Use a special radial artery catheter pack with small calibre needle,
  guide wire, and cannula
• Palpate the radial pulse
• Aim to cannulate proximal to the flexor skin creases to avoid the
  tough flexor retinaculum
• Advance the needle at 45° to the skin. As the artery is entered, blood
  flow is observed from the needle hub
• Other aspects of the cannulation follow the pattern of central venous
  line insertion
• Secure the cannula and attach a pressure monitoring line, transducer
  and flush facility.

Pericardiocentesis

Emergency drainage of the pericardial space is usually performed management of cardiac tamponade. When known or suspected nade has created a cardiac arrest situation, the procedure can and sh be performed as an immediate and potentially life-saving measure. other, less critical, cases echocardiography should be performed firs This investigation allows confirmation of the diagnosis and provides important information about the wisdom of and approach to pericardial aspiration.

Aspiration should only be attempted if there is a substantial fluid collection (>2 cm separation) between the pericardial layers at the access point of intended drainage. Following cardiac surgery or with certain chronic and infective aetiologies, there can be localised tamponade of a cardiac chamber, not amenable to percutaneous drainage. Obtain expert advice.

Imaging during the procedure is recommended. A cardiac catheterization laboratory is the ideal environment with radiographic screening and pressure monitoring, though echocardiographic imaging is increasingly used.

Procedure

- Position the patient at 45° to encourage pooling of the effusion at the inferior surface of the heart
- Prepared the skin and drape the patient in a sterile fashion
- Infiltrate local anaesthetic along the drainage track (passing just under the costal margin, following a line towards the tip of the left scapula)
- Conscious sedation may be required (e.g. midazolam)
- The skin incision point lies just below the xiphisternum. Use a scalpel blade to make a small incision to reduce skin friction for the passage of the drainage catheter
- Advance the needle, with syringe attached, maintaining negative pressure, and observe for the aspiration of fluid
- If echocardiography is used, agitated saline may be used to confirm the presence of the needle in the pericardial space
- Remove the syringe when fluid is obtained and advance the guidewire through the needle so that it loops in the cardiac shadow on X-ray screening or is visible in the pericardial space with echocardiography
- Remove the needle, leaving the guidewire in place
- Advance a dilator over the wire. Several passes may be required
- Advance the catheter over the wire and into the pericardial space
- Fluid can now be aspirated with a syringe
- Symptoms and haemodynamic compromise in tamponade will improve with removal of modest volumes of fluid (e.g. 20–50 mL)
- Samples are sent for biochemical, immunological, and microbiological analysis
- The drainage bag can then be connected, secured with sutures at the skin entry point and dressed with transparent occlusive dressings
- The catheter is usually left in situ for several hours to gauge the rate of drainage or reaccumulation (judged by echocardiography).

...ems of equipment

...mber of manufacturers now supply pericardial drainage packs.
- ...ong needle (15 cm) of at least 18 G calibre. A short bevel is an advantage to avoid potential cardiac laceration
- 'J' tip guidewire (0.035" diameter)
- Dilator (5–7 French)
- Pigtail or other drainage catheter with multiple distal side-holes
- Large calibre syringe for aspiration
- Drainage bag and connecting tubing.

Pericardiocentesis

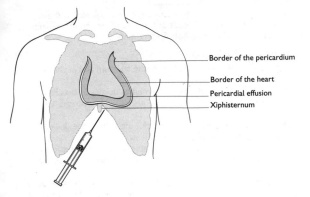

Border of the pericardium

Border of the heart

Pericardial effusion

Xiphisternum

Cardioversion/defibrillation

The quickest and most effective method of restoring sinus rhythm.

- Cardioversion is traditionally performed under sedation with intravenous benzodiazepines or under general anaesthesia (typically with propofol) according to hospital protocol
- Full resuscitation, airway management, external pacing facilities, and trained personnel should be immediately available
- Ensure that the patient is well oxygenated, starved for at least 4 hours (unless an emergency) and for elective procedures, patients should have signed a consent form
- As a minimum, monitoring should include indirect arterial oxygen saturation, blood pressure, and ECG monitoring
- Ensure the defibrillator electrodes are connected firmly to the machine, connect the ECG leads of the defibrillator to the patient and select a lead with the tallest QRS complex.

Ventricular arrhythmias

- Place gel electrode contact pads over the sternum and at the apex of the heart
- Defibrillation for VF should be performed as quickly as possible using unsynchronized high initial energies (200–360 J monophasic, 150–200 J biphasic)
- If defibrillation is repeatedly unsuccessful then check the device settings and consider a different defibrillator
- Cardioversion of haemodynamically stable VT is usually performed under sedation with intravenous benzodiazepines or with general anaesthesia
- If the patient is haemodynamically deteriorating it can be hazardous to delay treatment whilst awaiting an anaesthetist. Consider conscious sedation with IV midazolam (2–10 mg) or Diazemuls® (5–20 mg) ensuring close airway and respiratory monitoring
- Ensure the defibrillator is set to 'Synch.' so that the defibrillation shock is timed to coincide with the R wave. A dot should appear on the R wave of the ECG (and not the T wave). Use different leads if the synchronization is not optimal
- Typical starting energies for the cardioversion of VT are 200 J monophasic and 150 J biphasic.

rhythmias (AF and atrial flutter)

direct current (DC) cardioversion for AF has a success rate of
% for restoring sinus rhythm. Since as little as 5% of the energy
ered externally actually reaches the heart, high external energies
ve to be used. Monophasic defibrillators deliver energy in one direc-
on whereas modern biphasic devices deliver the energy wavefront
across the heart in two directions. The success rate for cardioversion
using a biphasic defibrillator is higher than for monophasic devices.

- For elective cardioversion, it is vital to know the patient's anticoagulation
  status before cardioversion. If the international normalized ratio (INR)
  has been greater than 2.0 for at least 4 weeks, the risk of thromboembolism for elective cardioversion of AF is less than 1%
- It is also useful to know the serum K^+ before defibrillation as
  hypokalaemia may precipitate early reinitiation of AF
- Place gel electrode contact pads over the sternum and at the apex
  of the heart
- Ensure the defibrillator is set to 'Synch.' so that the defibrillation shock
  is timed to coincide with the R wave. A dot should appear on the
  R wave of the ECG (and not the T wave). Use different leads if the
  synchronization is not optimal
- Higher initial energies are more likely to restore sinus rhythm for AF
  (360 J monophasic, 200 J biphasic). Lower energies (200 J, 150 J
  biphasic) are suitable for atrial flutter
- Firm pressure on the defibrillator electrodes (8–12 kg) significantly
  improves the cardioversion success rate by reducing thoracic
  impedance
- If sinus rhythm has not been restored after two shocks at maximum
  output consider changing the electrode position to anteroposterior by
  either rolling the patient onto their right side or by positioning an
  electrode plate behind the patient
- If sinus rhythm is still not restored after an anteroposterior shock then
  the patient should be recovered in the left lateral position and an
  alternative strategy obtained (internal cardioversion/drug facilitation)
  from a cardiologist (usually at a later date).

ECG recognition

Theory and principles 306
The current of injury 310
Bundle branch block (BBB) 314
ECG library 318
    Anterior myocardial infarction 319
    Inferior myocardial infarction 320
    Inferolateral-posterior myocardial infarction 321
    Myocardial ischaemia (LAD syndrome) 322
    Pericarditis 323
    Left bundle branch block 324
    Right bundle branch block 325
    Trifascicular block 326
    Junctional rhythm 327
    Second degree heart block (Mobitz I) 328
    Complete heart block 329
    Atrial fibrillation 330
    Pre-excited atrial fibrillation 331
    Atrial flutter 332
    Atrial tachycardia 333
    Supraventricular tachycardia (AVNRT) 334
    Supraventricular tachycardia (AVRT) 335
    Pre-excitation 336
    Ventricular tachycardia 337
    Accelerated idioventricular rhythm 338
    Long QT 339
    Brugada syndrome 340
    Arrhythmogenic right ventricular cardiomyopathy 341
    Pacemaker lead failure 342

Theory and principles

The art of ECG recognition

ECG interpretation is a fundamental art of medicine. When reading ECGs, basic principles are learnt and these are applied to each and every ECG encountered. Time and experience makes 'pattern recognition' possible. Combining both pattern recognition and fundamental principles is the cornerstone to the 'art of ECG recognition'. The following points will hopefully aid the reader to understand some aspects that are traditionally not well explained. The ECG recordings included hereafter will have salient features pointed out, and hopefully will act as an aid for pattern-recognition.

Key points

▶ The changing ECG should be regarded as the hallmark of ischaemic heart disease until proven otherwise.
▶ The diagnosis of ischaemia is not made on the ECG alone.
• An electrogram can be recorded from any site upon the body surface, however convention dictates a 12 different electrode configuration to produce what we know as the routine 12-lead ECG
• Other electrode configurations may be of use clinically (right ventricular electrodes, 📖 p.58, and posterior electrodes)
• An electrical wavefront moving towards an electrode appears as a positive deflection above the isoelectric line
• Each ECG lead 'looks at' a mean voltage of the entire electrical activity in the heart from a particular 'point of view':

ECG lead	Area that lead 'looks at'
Leads I & aVL	Lateral aspect of the whole myocardium.
Leads II, III & aVF	The inferior (caudal) aspect of the whole myocardium.
Lead aVR	Right lateral heart.
V1 & V2	Atria (with the right atrium moving towards these electrodes and the left atrium moving away) and the base of the ventricles.
V3 & V4	The septum and mid left ventricle.
V5 & V6	Left ventricle lateral wall and apex.

• An electrical wavefront moving away from an electrode appears as a negative deflection below the isoelectric line
• Hence, V1 which 'looks at' the base of the heart towards the right ventricle has a predominantly negative QRS, as the major vector of myocardial depolarization is away from that lead, towards the apex of the left ventricle
• V6, which 'looks at' the left ventricle apex, is correspondingly predominantly a strongly positive complex.

...al values

	milliseconds	small squares*
PR interval	0.12–0.2	3–5
QRS duration	≤0.12	Not >3
Axis	–30° to +120°	
QT interval	0.35–0.43[†]	9–11
P wave duration	<0.11	<3

* assuming paper speed of 25mm/second.
[†] must be corrected for heart rate and NB sex differences.

Mean frontal axis

- The chest leads (V1–V6) are not used
- Look at the most isoelectric complex—the axis will lie at 90° to this
- Look at the leads which are at 90° to the isoelectric lead—the most positive one will be close to the true axis, with the most negative lead being 180° to the axis
- Much has been made of the ECG axis, although in reality there are only a few important patterns to recognize:
  - RBBB & left or right axis deviation in bifascicular block
  - Left anterior hemiblock
  - 'Upward' or 'northward' axis of AV canal defects and often in fascicular ventricular tachycardia
  - Right axis deviation in right ventricular strain/overload, e.g. chest disease, including acute pulmonary embolism.

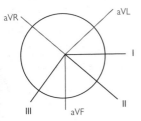

ECG lead vectors. The augmented leads (aVR, aVL and aVF) are spaced at 120°. The standard leads (I, II and III) are spaced at 60°.

Electrical conduction

- Electrical spread may be facilitated either by direct cell-to-cell depolarization (e.g. in the atria), or, as in the ventricles, via a specialized conduction system, termed the His–Purkinje system
- Cell-to-cell depolarization is relatively slow, producing more slurred, widened patterns of tracing (e.g. P waves, delta waves)
- His–Purkinje conduction is rapid, giving rise to the sharp deflections as normally seen in the QRS complex
- For example, in bundle branch block (📖 p.314), conduction through the ventricles is initially via the *His–Purkinje* system, and so begins as a sharp deflection in the QRS complex, followed by cell-to-cell depolarization which leads to QRS prolongation (>120 ms by definition in bundle branch block)
- In pre-excitation (📖 p.336) the ventricles are starting to depolarize via an anomalous ('accessory') pathway before the His–Purkinje system, thus the complex begins slurred before becoming sharper (depending upon the balance of activation between the accessory pathway and His–Purkinje system).

The origin of the waves of the ECG

- A single cardiac myocyte produces an electrical signal when it 'fires' (depolarizes), followed by another signal when it 'recovers' (repolarizes)
- The P wave represents atrial depolarization. It occurs from cell-to-cell, and thus is relatively slow in onset and duration giving a typical broad 'dome' shape
- The QRS wave is produced from depolarization via the His–Purkinje system. It is normally fast, and the whole of the right ventricle and left ventricle myocardium is depolarized in under 120 ms—hence the normal QRS duration of ≤120 ms
- The T wave represents ventricular repolarization ('resetting'). Thus measuring the onset of the QRS until the end of the T wave gives a measure of the time taken for ventricular myocytes to depolarize and repolarize ('fire and reset'). This is termed the QT interval.

...ation of accessory pathways on surface ECGs

..he acute management of patients with pre-excitation, accurate
..alization of the pathway is not necessary. It is important for
..lectrophysiologists, as it aids selection of the correct equipment and
approach to ablation (📖 p.336)
- However, there are some simple rules-of-thumb:
  - Dominant R wave V1 suggests left sided accessory pathways
    (i.e. looks more like RBBB because left heart is being stimulated
    prematurely over accessory pathway)
  - LBBB-like pattern suggests right sided accessory pathway
  - The negative delta wave 'points' to the accessory pathways position
    e.g. left free wall accessory pathways usually have negative delta
    wave in aVL, posteroseptal pathways (actually, inferiorly situated in
    true anatomy) have negative delta waves in II, III & aVF
  - As septal pathways move from posteroseptal, to mid-septal and
    anteroseptal, the delta wave tends to become more positive in the
    inferior leads in sequence—i.e. II, then aVF and then III
- Thus, in basic terms, AP localization may be simplified as follows:
  - Dominant R wave in V1? Yes—left sided. No—right sided
  - Negative delta wave in inferior leads? Yes—posteroseptal likely.
    No—free-wall likely.

Dominant R wave in V1

A useful tip for ECG interpretation is that a dominant R wave in lead V1
is usually associated with one of the following:
- RBBB
- Left sided accessory pathway
- Posterior MI
- Right ventricular hypertrophy
- Dextrocardia
- Infancy.

Reference
Fitzpatrick AP, Gonzales RP, Lesch MD et al. (1994). An algorithms for locating accessory pathways. *JACC* **23**(1), 107–116.

The current of injury

- A myocyte damaged by any cause (direct trauma, ischaemia) cannot regulate normal ionic transport. The earliest process to be affected is repolarization and thus the earliest changes seen on the ECG are usually in the ST segment of the ECG (i.e. the period at the very end of depolarization to repolarization)
- An injured myocyte produces an action potential which has a 'lower' (i.e. *more negative*) baseline. Taken as a group of cells, this gives the appearance of ST segment *elevation* when viewed from an electrode position directly adjacent to the damaged area
- In cardiac ischaemia (□ p.322), the endomyocardium becomes ischaemic first, as it is relatively less well perfused. The ST elevation is directed in an inward vector manifesting as ST segment depression when observed on surface electrodes
- In acute MI (□ p.319) the full thickness of myocardium is in jeopardy and so ST elevation is seen in those leads which 'look at' the affected territory (e.g. leads V1–6 in antero-septal infarcts, II, III and aVF in inferior infarcts)
- In left ventricular hypertrophy, the 'strain pattern' is believed to be a result of chronic subendocardial ischaemia due to the high metabolic demands of the increased muscle-mass and the diminished perfusion from high transmural pressures. Thus the cells may demonstrate chronic ST elevation which, when viewed on the surface ECG, manifest as non-dynamic ST depression. As it predominantly occurs in the left ventricle, it is typically seen in leads V4–6
- In temporary (and permanent) pacing (□ p.296), endomyocardial electrode contact is confirmed by a local signal of ST elevation obtained from the pacing-electrode tip. Conversely ST depression suggests penetration of the electrode through the ventricular wall into the pericardium.

atterns of **ST segment abnormalities**

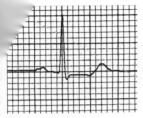

Typical, planar ST depression.

ST elevation due to MI.

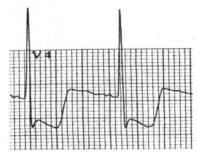

ST depression. This exaggerated response is often found in left ventricular hypertrophy and ischaemia—particularly during exercise tests. 'Strain' pattern can sometimes be this severe, especially in severe aortic stenosis and hypertrophic cardiomyopathy.

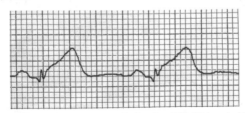

'Hyper-acute' ST changes. Often this is the first sign of ST shift in acute MI. It may also be seen in hyper-adrenergic states, including subarachnoid haemorrhage and post arrest (especially after epinephrine has been given) where it does not necessarily represent infarction.

True posterior myocardial infarction

- Differentiating between true posterior MI and ischaemic ST depre.
  may be difficult
- The key is to look at the 'shape' of the ST elevation from a posterior
  point of view using either true posterior leads or holding the ECG up
  to the light and looking at V1–3 reversed (i.e. from behind, upside
  down)
- The following figures show (left) V1–3 in standard fashion, with (right)
  the leads reversed, such that V3 is uppermost
- The pattern in reversed V1 (lowermost complex, right panel) looks
  like typical ST elevation.

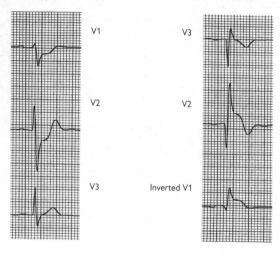

Bundle branch block (BBB)

The bundle of His exits the AV node within the inter-ventricular se
and bifurcates into the left and right bundle branches. The left bu
sub-divides further into the left posterior and anterior fascicles.
bundles can develop conduction block from a variety of sources, bo
transient and permanent. Characteristic changes may then be observec
on the ECG.

Left bundle branch block (LBBB) 🕮 p.324

- Activation proceeds through the bundle of His and into the right
  bundle as normal, activating the right ventricle early. This is rapid, and
  hence there is a sharp deflection initially
- Septal and left ventricular activation is delayed, hence the QRS con-
  figuration is almost as it would be in normal activation but 'wider'
- As septal depolarization is reversed (now occurring from right to left)
  there is an initial Q wave in V1 and an R–S–R pattern in V6—i.e. V1 is
  W shaped and V6 is M shaped
- In true LBBB there can be no initial Q wave in 'left-looking' leads, V5,
  V6 and I, no matter how small the deflection.

Clinical significance of LBBB

- Almost always associated with organic heart disease (e.g. ischaemia,
  cardiomyopathy, conduction tissue disease, hypertensive heart disease,
  infiltration)
- ST elevation is very difficult to interpret and thus cannot be relied
  upon to diagnose acute myocardial infarction.

▶ New onset LBBB with ischaemic sounding chest pain is supportive of
acute MI and thus is considered an indication for reperfusion therapy
🕮 p.52.

Right bundle branch block (RBBB) 🕮 p.325

- Right ventricular activation occurs via the left bundle branch and thus
  is delayed
- The interventricular septum is depolarized in the normal fashion (left
  to right)
- Because the right ventricular is activated just after the left ventricle it
  typically produces an R–S–R pattern in V1 (M shape)
- In V6 it may produce a deep S wave, giving a modified W type pattern,
  although often this is not apparent. The changes in V1 are much more
  constant.

Clinical significance of RBBB

- May be normal, especially in young and the fit
- May be a sign of right heart strain, e.g. acute PE, right ventricular
  overload due to shunts
- Often seen in atrial septal defects, with right axis deviation in atrial
  septal type ('secundum') defects and left/upright axis in AV canal
  defects ('primum')

am & Marrow'

- ...iam and Marrow are often used aide memoirs to recognize and ...ferentiate LBBB and RBBB respectively
- The first letter of each word refers to the appearance of the QRS complex in V1 and the last letter in V6
- The double letters in the middle give the type of BBB. In practice, 'WiLLiaM' for LBBB tends to work quite well as a rule of thumb, but as mentioned above, 'MaRRoW' for RBBB tends to fall down because V6 often does not look like an M shape.

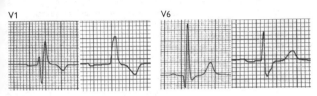

Left: V1 in two cases of **RBBB**, and right, V6. The 'MaRRoW' principle can only be interpreted with a degree of 'artistic licence'.

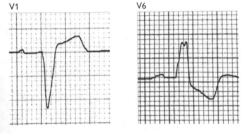

V1 (left panel) and V6 (right) in **LBBB**. Again, applying the 'WiLLiaM' principle requires a little imagination.

Alternating LBBB/RBBB
- A sign of bifascicular block
- In the presence of unexplained syncope, transient higher degrees of AV block should be considered.

Bifascicular and trifascicular block
- Conduction delay, usually due to widespread fibrotic disease is present within the AV node, His bundle, and bundle branches
- Left anterior hemiblock usually results in left axis deviation
- Left posterior hemiblock usually results in right axis deviation
- Trifascicular block is a misnomer, as it really represents conduction delay. Logically, if all three fascicles were actually blocked there would be complete heart block
- Bifascicular block is most commonly seen with RBBB and left anterior hemiblock. Hence there is RBBB and left axis deviation
- In trifascicular block, the classic ECG shows 1° heart block, RBBB and left axis deviation (📖 p.326)
- In an asymptomatic patient with trifascicular block permanent pacing is not indicated. In the presence of unexplained syncope however a bradycardic cause is likely
- Risk of complete heart block (may be transient) is 2–6% per annum, with asymptomatic patients forming the lower percentage, and those with unexplained syncope the higher.

BBB and cardiac catheterization
- Direct trauma to a bundle may produce BBB (usually transient)—so-called 'mechanical bundle block', this may last for several hours or even days
- In pre-existing BBB, catheter-based procedures on the contralateral side may produce complete heart block, with acute compromise. This occurs most typically during right heart procedures with pre-existing LBBB (e.g. Swan–Ganz lines, pacing, etc.).

Paced complexes and VT morphology
- Pacing from the right ventricular apex causes the septum and left ventricle to be activated right to left, rather like LBBB. Thus paced complexes have the LBBB 'WiLLiaM' type morphology. In left ventricular pacing (as part of cardiac resynchronization therapy) the pure left ventricular paced complex has RBBB morphology
- For similar reasons, VT with LBBB type morphology may be exiting within the right heart, and RBBB morphologies may be exiting within the left heart.

...ndle branch block and SVT rate

When a BBB develops during SVT it is often labelled a 'rate-related' BBB. However, careful attention should be paid to the tachycardia rate. If the rate or cycle-length actually slows, then an accessory pathway ipsilateral to the block is implicated—i.e. LBBB with slowing implicates a left free wall accessory pathway, and RBBB suggests a right sided accessory pathway. The mechanism is due to the extra time the head of the re-entrant wave takes to cross the septum after it leaves the AV node and spreads through the His–Purkinje system.

Example: In AVRT with a left sided free-wall accessory pathway, the circuit travels down the AV node, through both left and right ventricles, before climbing the accessory pathway back into the left atrium, and so on. If LBBB develops, the wavefront must travel down the right bundle, across the septum and into the left ventricle using cell-to-cell spread. This adds about 40–60 milliseconds to its journey and results in an increase in tachycardia cycle length by the same amount.

V1   V6

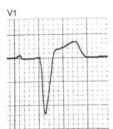 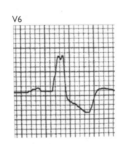

Paced rhythm from right ventricular apex, with V1 (left) and V6 (right) shown. Depolarization initiating from the RV apex 'mimics' to a certain degree, LBBB, as reflected in the tracings above. RBBB-paced patterns are due to inadvertent left ventricular capture via an ASD/PFO, VSD or coronary sinus branch. With a bi-ventricular pacemaker it may represent a left ventricular lead or programming problems.

ECG library

The following collection of ECGs is presented to act as a reminder of t
12-lead ECG patterns of common (and a few uncommon) cardiac conditions.

Anterior myocardial infarction

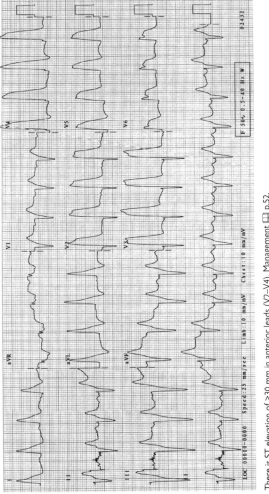

There is ST elevation of >30 mm in anterior leads (V2–V4). Management 📖 p.52.

Inferior myocardial infarction

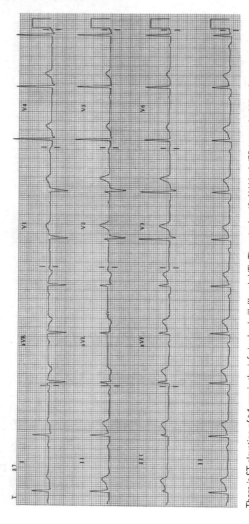

There is ST elevation of >1 mm in the inferior leads (II, III and aVF). There is also 1° AV block (PR interval >200 ms). Management ⮌ p.52.

Inferolateral-posterior myocardial infarction

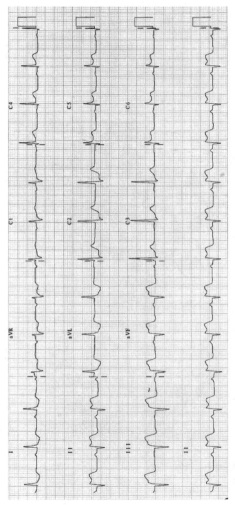

There is ST elevation of >1 mm in the inferior leads (II, III and aVF) and lateral leads (V5 and V6) with ST depression in V1 and V2. The R wave in V1 is dominant. Management □ p.52.

Myocardial ischaemia (LAD syndrome)

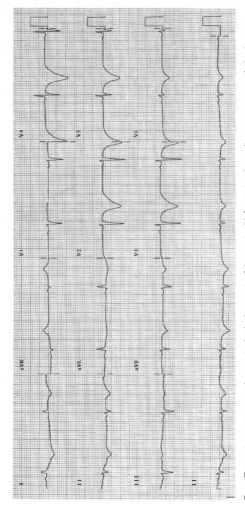

Deep T wave inversion across the anterior leads. A stenosis of the proximal left anterior descending coronary artery lesion is commonly the culprit. Management 🕮 p.62.

Pericarditis

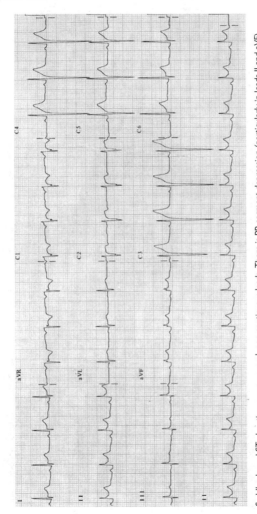

Saddle-shaped ST elevation across several, non-contiguous leads. There is PR segment depression (particularly in leads II and aVF).
Management ☐ p.183.

Left bundle branch block

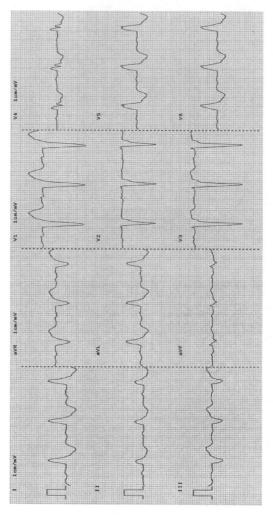

LBBB. Broad QRS complex with a Q wave in V1 ('W'shape) and RSR pattern in V6 ('M'shape). 🔲 p.314.

Right bundle branch block

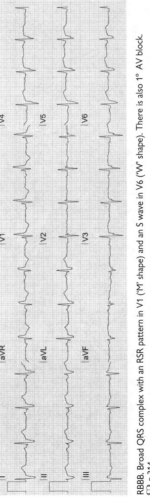

RBBB. Broad QRS complex with an RSR pattern in V1 ('M' shape) and an S wave in V6 ('W' shape). There is also 1° AV block.
📖 p.314.

Trifascicular block

There is right bundle branch block, 1° AV block and left anterior hemiblock (left axis deviation). 📖 p.316.

Junctional rhythm

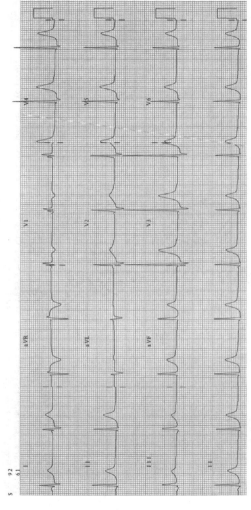

P waves are seen before the first complex but then are buried within the QRS complex. ☐ p.130.

Second degree heart block (Mobitz I)

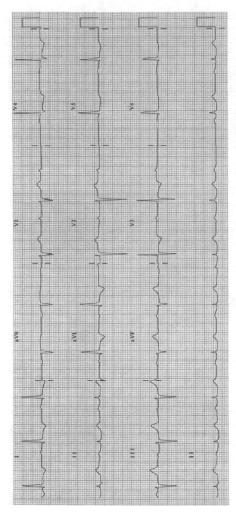

There is progressive lengthening of the PR interval until a P wave is non-conducted and a QRS is dropped (Wenckebach). The PR interval after the dropped beat is the shortest. 📖 p.132.

Complete heart block

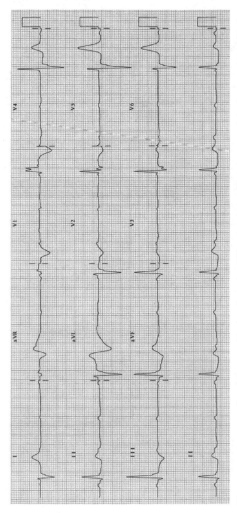

There are regular non-conducted P waves with a broad complex QRS escape rhythm. There is no association between the atrial and the ventricular rates. Management ☐ p.133.

Atrial fibrillation

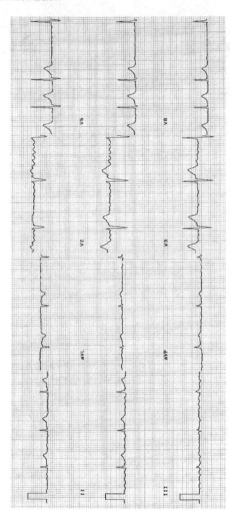

Irregularly irregular ventricular rhythm with no discernible P waves. Management ☐ p.140.

e-excited atrial fibrillation

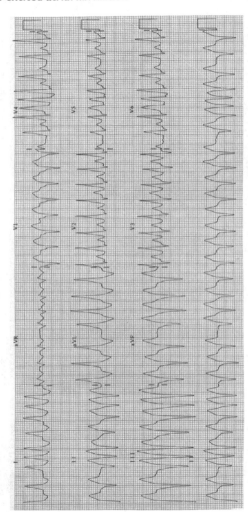

An irregular broad complex tachycardia with very rapid ventricular activation and conduction. Management □ p.143.

Atrial flutter

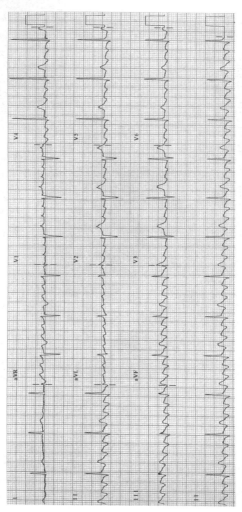

The baseline is irregular with a 'saw-tooth' pattern. The flutter waves are conducted with a 4:1 pattern to the ventricle.
Management 📖 p.144.

Atrial tachycardia

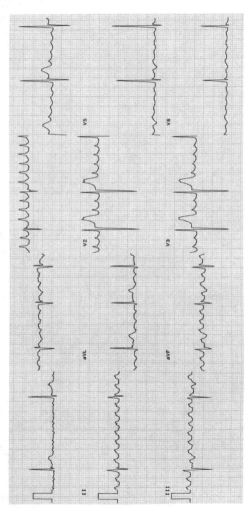

The baseline is irregular with very rapid atrial activation (300 bpm) and a positive P wave in V1 suggesting a focal atrial tachycardia. The baseline returns to normal between each atrial beat. Management ▯ p.148.

Supraventricular tachycardia (AVNRT)

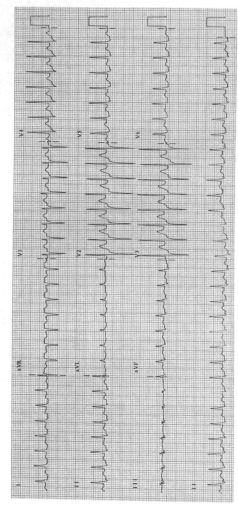

A narrow complex tachycardia. The terminal deflection upon the R wave of the complexes of V1 are likely to represent the R-prime (R') sign. R' suggests a terminal portion of P wave is inscribed there. With a ventricular-to-atrial conduction time so short, AVNRT is the most likely diagnosis. Management 📖 p.150.

Supraventricular tachycardia (AVRT)

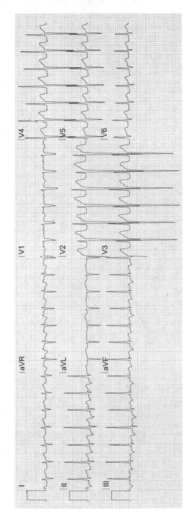

A narrow complex tachycardia. There is retrograde P wave activation (clearly seen in V1 before the QRS complex). Management 📖 p.152.

Pre-excitation

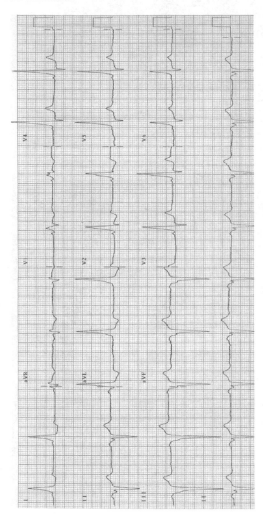

Short PR interval due to the presence of a delta wave. There is a RBBB-type pattern present, suggesting the accessory pathway is left sided. The negative delta waves inferiorly suggest that the accessory pathway is posteroseptal. Management 🕮 p.152.

Ventricular tachycardia

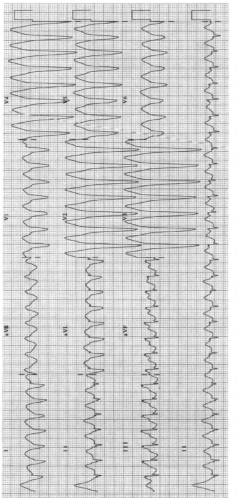

A broad complex tachycardia with a ventricular rate of 180 bpm. AV dissociation is seen with buried P waves in V6. There is concordance across the chest leads. Management ◻ p.156.

Accelerated idioventricular rhythm

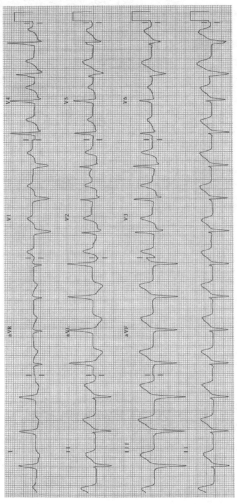

An automatic ventricular rhythm with a rate <100 bpm. Usually seen in the context of myocardial ischaemia or infarction.

Long QT

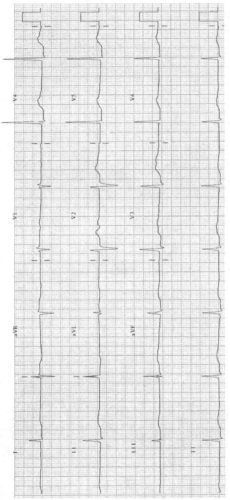

The QT interval (start of the Q wave to the end of the T wave) is prolonged (>600 ms). 📖 p.160.

Brugada syndrome

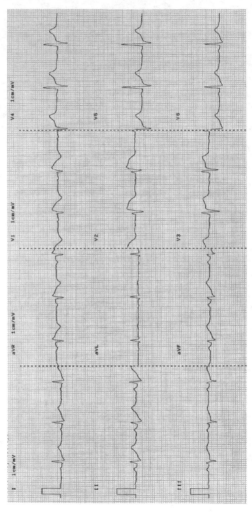

Right precordial ST elevation with T wave inversion in V1–V3. Association with sudden cardiac death. 📖 p.34.

Arrhythmogenic right ventricular cardiomyopathy

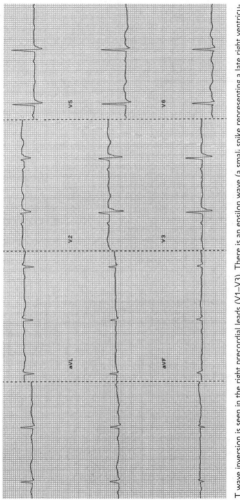

T wave inversion is seen in the right precordial leads (V1–V3). There is an epsilon wave (a small spike representing a late right ventricular potential) seen in V1 and V2 in the upstroke of the ST segment. Associated with VT. 📖 p.156.

Pacemaker lead failure

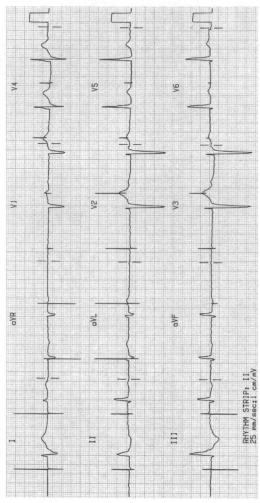

RHYTHM STRIP: II
25 mm/sec;1 cm/mV

Pacemaker spikes can be seen with no ventricular capture. The ventricular lead had displaced.

Index

A

accelerated idioventricular rhythm 338
ACE inhibitors 70, 241
acute coronary syndromes 45–66
  classification 47
  definition 46
  non-ST elevation myocardial infarction 62–5
  pathophysiology 46–7
  ST elevation myocardial infarction 48
acute heart failure 67–85
  aetiology 69
  causes of decompensation 68
  clinical features 68
  continuing management 70, 73
  differential diagnosis 70
  goals of therapy 74
  haemodynamic profiles 71
  immediate management 70, 73
  investigation 68
  monitoring 74
  systolic vs. diastolic 69
acute thoracic syndromes 178–9
  intramural haematoma 178
  penetrating atherosclerotic ulcer 178
adenosine 137
adrenaline (epinephrine) 9–12
Advanced Life Support algorithm 5
alteplase 54
amiodarone 166
amlodipine overdose 265
amoxicillin 103
amphetamine overdose 272
angina pectoris 16, 18, 19, 46–7
  Canadian Cardiovascular Society classification 255
  peri-operative issues 254

  unstable see unstable angina
anti-cancer drugs 270
anticoagulation
  Eisenmenger syndrome 238
  peri-operative issues 256
  in pregnancy 216
  prosthetic valves 109
aortic coarctation 226–7
aortic disease in pregnancy 210
aortic dissection 19, 56, 170–5
  antihypertensive therapy 174
  causes and associations 170
  clinical signs 170
  complications 174
  differential diagnosis 56
  follow-up 175
  hypertensive emergencies 279
  imaging 171
  investigations 171
  pharmacological management 172
  presentation 170
  prognosis 175
  Stanford classification 171
  surgical management 174
  thoracic 16
aortic regurgitation 34, 77, 91, 114, 115
  eponymous signs in 115
  peri-operative issues 256
  in pregnancy 212
aortic stenosis 34, 77, 91, 112–13
  acute problems 112
  causes 112
  clinical features 112
  peri-operative issues 254–257, 256
  in pregnancy 212
  treatment 112
aortography 171
arrhythmias 287–303, 29
  atrial fibrillation 84, 116, 137, 140–3
  atrial flutter 145, 137, 144–7
  atrial tachycardia 137, 148–9

atrioventricular block 132–4
atrioventricular nodal reentrant tachycardia 150–1
atrioventricular reentrant tachycardia 152–3
  bradycardia 126
  congenital 239
  electrical storms 162
  junctional bradycardia 130–1
  monomorphic ventricular tachycardia 156–8
  peri-operative issues 255
  in pregnancy 213
  sinus arrest 128
  sinus bradycardia 126–7
  sinus tachycardia 138–9
  supraventricular tachycardia 317, 334
  tachycardia 136–7
  treatment 166
  ventricular fibrillation 154
  ventricular tachycardia see ventricular tachycardia
arrhythmogenic right ventricular cardiomyopathy 341
arterial line, insertion of 298
atrial fibrillation 116, 137, 140–3
  and atrioventricular block 134
  cardioversion/defibrillation 303
  electrocardiogram 330, 331
  and heart failure 84
  management 143
  post-operative 259
  pre-excited 143
  in pregnancy 213
  with severe haemodynamic compromise 142
atrial flutter 145, 137, 144–7
  cardioversion/defibrillation 303
  congenital 239
  electrocardiogram 332

atrial flutter (Continued)
management 147
in pregnancy 213
with severe haemodynamic compromise 137, 144
atrial septal defect 220–1
atrial switch operation 242–5
atrial tachycardia 137, 148–9
electrocardiogram 333
atrioventricular block 132–4
and atrial fibrillation/flutter 134
and myocardial infarction 58, 134
atrioventricular conduction block 259
atrioventricular nodal reentrant tachycardia 150–1
atrioventricular reentrant tachycardia 152–3, 213, 239
atrioventricular septal defect 224, 225

B

balloon valvuloplasty 116
bendroflumethiazide 71
Bentall operation 242–5
benzylpenicillin 103
beta-blockers 70, 241
and heart failure 84
overdose 264
prophylactic perioperative 255
bifascicular block 316
Blalock-Taussig shunt 242–5
bradycardia 126
junctional 130–1
sinus 126–7
brain natriuretic peptide 69
breathlessness 21–26
causes 23
diagnosis 22–3
investigations 24
Brock procedure 242–5
bronchoconstriction 76
Brugada syndrome 34
electrocardiogram 340
bundle branch block 314–17
alternating 316
bifascicular and trifascicular 316
and cardiac catheterization 316
electrocardiogram 341, 324, 325

left 314, 315
paced complexes and VT morphology 316
right 314, 315
and supraventricular tachycardia 317, 334
William & Marrow 315

C

calcium channel blocker overdose 265
cardiac arrest 4
cardiac arrhythmia see arrhythmias
cardiac asthma 76
cardiac catheterization 316
cardiac surgery 258–9
cardiac syncope 34
cardiac tumours 282–3
clinical features 282
lymphoma 283
metastatic 283
myxoma 282
papillary fibroelastomas 282
sarcomas 283
cardiogenic shock 58, 78–9, 85
cardiomyopathies 80–3
arrhythmogenic right ventricular 341
dilated 82
hypertrophic 34, 80
restrictive 82
cardiorenal syndrome 76
cardiotoxic drug overdose 17
amphetamine 272
anti-cancer drugs 270
beta-blockers 264
calcium channel blockers 265
cocaine 272
digoxin 266–7
ecstasy 273
information sources 262
management 262
QT prolongation 274–5
theophylline 269
tricyclic antidepressants 268
cardiovascular collapse 4–5
diagnosis 6
immediate actions 8–9
initial assessment 6–7
investigation and treatment 10
cardioversion 215, 302–3
carotid sinus massage 33
carotid sinus syndrome 32

central venous lines 11, 290–3
choice of approach 290
femoral vein approach 293
internal jugular approach 171, 291
subclavian approach 292
central venous pressure 11
chest pain 15–20
associated physical signs 18
causes 17
diagnosis 16
investigations 19
presentation 16–17
chest X-ray
pulmonary embolism 192
pulmonary hypertension 196
valve disease 111
chronic valve disease 94
circulatory management 8, 10
cocaine overdose 272
hypertensive emergencies 279
commotio cordis 280
complete heart block 58, 132–4
computed tomography, aortic dissection 171
conduction disorders, perioperative issues 256
congenital heart disease 15
aortic coarctation 226–7
arrhythmias 239
atrial septal defect 220–1
atrioventricular septal defect 224, 225
cyanosis 236, 237
Eisenmenger syndrome 238
heart failure 240
patent ductus arteriosus 224–5
single ventricle 234–5, 243
surgical procedures 242–5
syncope 240
tetralogy of Fallot 232–3
transposition of great arteries 228–9, 230–1
ventricular septal defect 76, 222–3
constrictive pericarditis 186
continuous positive airway pressure 10
coronary angiography, aortic dissection 171
coronary artery
anatomy 50

...ry artery bypass
...afting 64, 252, 258–9
...onary artery disease,
  peri-operative issues 254
coronary atherothrombosis
  46
coronary revascularization
  252
  peri-operative issues 254
Corrigan's sign 115
current of injury 310–12
cyanosis 236, 237
  management 237
  multi-organ consequences
    237

D

D-dimer assay 192
Damus-Kaye-Stansel opera-
  tion 242–5
de Musset's sign 115
defibrillation 215, 302–3
diabetes mellitus 46, 56, 76
digoxin 71, 166, 241
digoxin overdose 266–7
  clinical features 266
  investigations 266
  management 266
  poor prognostic
    indicators 267
  predisposing factors
    267
dilated cardiomyopathy 82
diltiazem overdose 265
diuretics 81
  loop 71, 241
  non-loop 71
dobutamine 9–12
dopamine 9–12
Dressler syndrome 60
driving
  myocardial infarction 60
  syncope 31
Duke criteria (modified) for
  diagnosis of infective
  endocarditis 101
Duroziez's sign 115

E

echocardiography 89, 99
  endocarditis 100
  intra-cardiac 204
  paradoxical emboli 204,
    205
  prosthetic valves 106
  pulmonary embolism 192
  pulmonary hypertension
    196
  saline contrast 204
  systemic emboli 203

transoesophageal 171,
  173, 203
transthoracic 171, 203
valve disease 111
ecstasy overdose 273
Eisenmenger syndrome 238
electrical storms 162
electrocardiogram 20, 30
  24-hour monitoring 28,
    40
  accelerated idioventricular
    rhythm 338
  accessory pathways 309
  ambulatory monitoring
    40
  arrhythmogenic right
    ventricular cardio-
    myopathy 341
  atrial fibrillation 330, 331
  atrial flutter 332
  atrial tachycardia 333
  Brugada syndrome 340
  bundle branch block 341,
    314–17, 324, 325
  chest pain 63
  current of injury 310–12
  dominant R wave in V1
    301
  electrical conduction 308
  heart block 328, 329
  hypertrophic cardio-
    myopathy 81
  junctional rhythm 327
  lead vectors 307
  left bundle branch block
    314, 324
  long QT syndrome 339
  mean frontal axis 307
  myocardial infarction 49,
    51, 312, 319, 320, 321
  myocardial ischaemia 322
  normal values 307, 306–9
  pacemaker lead failure
    342
  pericarditis 323
  pre-excitation 336
  pulmonary embolism 192,
    193
  pulmonary hypertension
    196, 199
  second degree heart
    block 328
  supraventricular
    tachycardia 334, 335
  theory and principles
    306–9
  trifascicular block 326
  valve disease 111
  ventricular tachycardia
    337
  wave origins 309
embolus
  paradoxical 204

pulmonary 16, 18, 19,
  190–5
systemic 202–3
endocarditis see infective
  endocarditis
endovascular aortic stenting
  174
ephedrine 9–12
epinephrine (adrenaline)
  9–12
esmolol 174, 166
extrinsic cardiogenic
  shock 7

F

flecainide 166
flucloxacillin 103
Fontan operation 236, 242–5

G

gastro-oesophageal reflux
  17, 39
gentamicin 103
Glenn shunt 243
glyceryl trinitrate 9–12
glycoprotein IIb/IIIa
  inhibition 64

H

heart block
  complete 58
  electrocardiogram 328,
    329
  second degree 328
heart failure
  acute see acute heart
    failure and atrial
    fibrillation 84
  aemodynamic profiles 71
  congenital heart disease
    240
  peri-operative issues 255
  pregnancy 210
  and sepsis 84
  treatment 241
heart murmurs 91
  aortic regurgitation 34,
    77, 91, 114, 115
  aortic stenosis 34, 77, 91,
    112–13
  grading 91
  infective endocarditis 99
  innocent 91
  mitral regurgitation 59,
    91, 118–19
  mitral stenosis 91, 116
  see also valve disease
Holter monitor (24 hour
  ECG monitor) 32, 40

hypertension
 peri-operative issues 255
 in pregnancy 214–15
hypertensive crisis 76
hypertensive emergencies
 278–9
 clinical signs 278
 investigations 278
 management 278
 presentation 278
hypertrophic cardio-
 myopathy 34, 80
hypotension 58
 post-operative 258

I

implantable cardioverter
 defibrillators 154, 164
 peri-operative issues 257
infective endocarditis
 96–104
 clinical features 98
 complications 104
 culture negative 104
 diagnosis 100
 echocardiography 99
 heart murmurs in 99
 investigations 100
 modified Duke criteria
 101
 peri-operative issues 257
 presentation 98
 prophylaxis 96, 97, 257
 risk 97
 treatment 102, 103
inotropes 9–12
intra-aortic balloon counter
 pulsation 12, 13
intramural haematoma 178
intrinsic cardiogenic shock 7

J

Jatene procedure 242–5
Jones criteria for acute
 rheumatic fever 111
junctional bradycardia
 130–1
junctional rhythm 327

K

Killip class 57
Konno operation 244
Kussmaul's sign 18

L

labetalol 174
Lecompte manoeuvre 244

left ventricular aneurysm 60
left ventricular impairment
 69, 34, 58, 80, 82, 84, 85,
 94
 see also heart failure
lidocaine 166
long QT syndrome 34,
 160–1, 274–5
 electrocardiogram 339
loop diuretics 71, 241

M

magnesium sulphate 166
magnetic resonance imag-
 ing, aortic dissection
 171, 173
Marfan syndrome 176, 210
metaraminal 9–12
mitral prolapse 119
mitral regurgitation 59, 91,
 118–19
 acute problems 118
 causes 118
 clinical features 118
 mitral prolapse 119
 myocardial infarction 59
 peri-operative issues 256
 in pregnancy 212
 surgery 119
mitral stenosis 91, 116
 peri-operative issues 256
 in pregnancy 212
mitral valve rupture 76
mixed aortic valve disease
 114–15
Mobitz second degree heart
 block 132, 133
monoamine oxidase inhibi-
 tors 279
monomorphic ventricular
 tachycardia 156–8
morphine 71
Müller's sign 115
Mustard operation 244
myocardial infarction 49
 and atrioventricular block
 134
 and cardiogenic shock 85
 complications 58–61
 differential diagnosis 56
 discharge medication 60
 electrocardiogram 49, 51,
 312, 319, 320, 321
 non-ST elevation 62–5
 peri-operative issues 254
 post-infarct management
 60
 in pregnancy 211
 prognostic indicators 57
 risk stratification and
 prognosis 56, 57

ST elevation 48
 thrombolysis 54
myocardial ischaemia 32
myocarditis 79

N

National Confidential
 Enquiry into Perio-
 operative Death 248
neurally-mediated (reflex)
 syncope 29
neurally-mediated (vasovagal) syncope 32
nifedipine overdose 265
nitrates 71
non-cardiogenic shock 7
non-invasive ventilation 10
non-loop diuretics 71
non-ST elevation myo-
 cardial infarction 62–5
noradrenaline 9–12
Norwood operation 244

O

oesophageal pain 17
orthopnoea 68
orthostatic hypotension 29,
 32–3

P

pacemakers 126, 128, 133,
 134
 lead failure 342
 overdrive pacing 161
 peri-operative issues 257
palpitation 37–42
 causes 39
 definition 38
 diagnosis 38–9
 general management 40
 investigations 40
paradoxical emboli 204,
 205
patent ductus arteriosus
 224–5
penetrating atherosclerotic
 ulcer 178
percutaneous coronary
 intervention 52
peri-operative care 16
 cardiac surgery 258–9
 coronary revascularization
 252
 determining risk 252
 predictors of risk 250–1
 pre-operative assessment
 248
 specific conditions 254–7
pericardial effusion 185

pericardial tamponade 184–5
pericardiocentesis 300–1
  equipment 301
  procedure 300, 301
pericarditis 17, 18, 19, 56, 59, 182–3
  causes 182
  clinical signs 182
  constrictive 186
  diagnosis 183
  electrocardiogram 323
  investigations 183
  management 183
  peri-operative issues 254
  presentation 182
peri-operative risk prediction 250–1
  anaesthetic factors 251
  patient factors 250
  surgery factors 251
phaeochromocytoma 279
polymorphic ventricular tachycardia 160–1
post-pericardiotomy syndrome 259
Pott's anastomosis shunt 244
pre-excitation (Wolff-Parkinson-White syndrome) 152–3
  with AF, treatment 143
  electrocardiogram 336
pregnancy 14
  anticoagulation 216
  aortic disease 210
  arrhythmias 213
  cardiac issues 208, 209
  cardioversion 215
  clinical indicators of pathological states 208
  heart failure 210
  hypertension 214–5
  myocardial infarction 211
  normal physiological changes 208
  pulmonary embolism 211
  valvular heart disease 212
pre-operative assessment 248
procainamide 166
procedures 19
  cardioversion/defibrillation 302–3
  central venous lines 290–3
  general considerations 288
  insertion of arterial line 298
  pericardiocentesis 300–1
  pulmonary artery catheters 294–5
  temporary pacing 296–7
propranolol 174

prosthetic valves 106–9
  anticoagulation 109
  complications 108
  echocardiography 106
protein losing enteropathy 236
pulmonary angiography 195
pulmonary artery catheters 294–5
  normal ranges 295
pulmonary embolism 16, 18, 19, 190–5
  investigations 192
  management 194
  in pregnancy 211
  presentation and signs 190
  risk factors 191
pulmonary hypertension 196
  classification and causes 197
  investigations 196, 199
  management 198
  presentation 196
pulmonary oedema 58, 85
  intractable 76
  non-cardiogenic 71
pulmonary regurgitation 120–1
pulmonary stenosis 120, 121

Q

Quincke's sign 115

R

Rastelli operation 244
reinfarction 59
reperfusion therapy 52–6
  indications for 54
respiratory failure 23
respiratory management in collapsed patients 8
restrictive cardiomyopathy 82
rheumatic fever 110–11
  diagnosis 111
  presentation 110
  prevention of recurrence 110
  treatment 110
  valve disease 111
rifampicin 103
right heart catheterization 295
right heart failure 76
right ventricular infarction 58
risk factors
  infective endocarditis 97
  pulmonary embolism 191
Ross operation 244

S

saline contrast echo-cardiography 204, 205
Senning operation 245
sepsis 84
shock 4–5
  cardiogenic 58, 78–9, 85
  causes 7
  see also cardiovascular collapse
single ventricle 234–5, 243
  Fontan operation 236
sinus arrest 128
sinus bradycardia 126–7
sinus tachycardia 39, 137, 138–9
sodium nitroprusside 174, 71
spironolactone 241
ST elevation myocardial infarction 48
Stanford classification of aortic dissection 171
streptokinase 54
subarachnoid haemorrhage 279
supraventricular tachycardia 39, 152–3, 317, 334
  bundle branch block 317, 334
  congenital heart disease 239
  electrocardiogram 334, 335
syncope 04, 80, 128, 133
  aortic stenosis 112–13
  causes 29
  congenital heart disease 240
  definition 28
  diagnosis 28–9
  investigations 30–1
systemic emboli 202–3
  causes 203
  investigations 202
  management 202
  presentation 202

T

tachycardia 136–7
  atrial 137, 148–9
  atrioventricular nodal reentrant 150–1
  atrioventricular reentrant tachycardia 152–3, 213, 239
  monomorphic ventricular 156–9
  sinus 138–9
  supraventricular 334, 317
  ventricular see ventricular tachycardia

temporary pacing 126, 128, 133, 134, 296–7
  configuring pacemaker settings 297
  external (transcutaneous) temporary pacing 296
  transvenous temporary pacemaker insertion 296
  wire position 297
tenecteplase 54
tetralogy of Fallot 232–3
theophylline overdose 269
thromboembolism 236
thrombolysis 54, 194
  contraindications 55
thrombophilia screen 192
thyrotoxicosis 39, 76
tilt-table testing 32
TIMI risk score 65
tissue perfusion 85
torsade de pointes 160–1, 274–5
transoesophageal echocardiography
  aortic dissection 171, 173
  systemic emboli 203
transposition of great arteries 228–9, 230–1
  arterial switch operation 228
  atrial switch operation 228
transthoracic echocardiography
  aortic dissection 171
  systemic emboli 203
Traube's sign 115
Trauma (cardiac) 280
  blunt cardiac trauma 280
  penetrating cardiac trauma 280

tricuspid regurgitation 122
tricuspid stenosis 122
tricyclic antidepressant overdose 268
trifascicular block 316
  electrocardiogram 326
troponin 51, 55
  in pericarditis 183
Turner syndrome 210

U

unstable angina 62–5
  glycoprotein IIb/IIIa inhibition 64
  immediate management 62
  investigations 62
  recent percutaneous coronary intervention 64
  risk stratification and early invasive treatment 64
  signs 62
  symptoms 62
  TIMI risk score 65

V

valve disease 87–123
  acute problems 88–95
  chronic 94
  investigations 89
  management 90
  peri-operative issues 256
  in pregnancy 212
  presentation 89
  rheumatic fever 111
  surgery 92–box
  see also individual valves

valve replacement 92–box
  in infective endocarditis 102
  prosthetic valves 106–9
vancomycin 103
vasodilators 71, 198
ventricular arrhythmia 58
  cardioversion/defibrillation 302
ventricular fibrillation 154
ventricular septal defect 76, 222–3
  myocardial infarction 59
  operated patients 222
  restrictive and non-restrictive 223
  unoperated patients 222
ventricular septal rupture 59
ventricular tachycardia 60, 137, 156
  congenital 239
  electrocardiogram 337
  management 158
  monomorphic 156–8
  overdrive pacing 161
  polymorphic (torsade de pointes) 160–1
  in pregnancy 213
verapamil 166
  overdose 265

W

Waterston shunt 245
Wenckebach phenomenon 133
Wolff–Parkinson–White syndrome (see pre-excitation)

:☺: —A true emergency, as outlined above. Memorizing these conditions may help, rather than referring to this book when the patient is in the department! Call for immediate senior help. Try to remain calm and quickly assess the ABCs. Once the problem has been dealt with, remember to re-assess—other problems may have been forgotten or missed in the heat of the moment.

:☺: —These patients still need to be assessed very quickly, but you do not need to drop everything and run (so long as their ABCs have been managed). These patients can quickly shift into the emergency category if not sorted soon. Consider senior help/advise.

① —The majority of patients will fall into this and the last category. Although they do not need to be seen straight away, make sure you assess them thoroughly—some conditions can deteriorate if not treated properly. Think carefully of potential complications that may develop, such as atrioventricular block with inferior MIs or tamponade with pericardial effusions. Liaise with specialist help, if necessary.

⑦ —These are non urgent conditions and general points of interest. Many of these patients, strictly speaking, should not come to casualty in the first place.